MY LIFE WITH AUTISM

Michael Feldman

Published by New Generation Publishing in 2020

First Edition

Paperback ISBN: 978-1-80031-613-3
Hardback ISBN: 978-1-80031-612-6

I have tried to recreate events, locales and conversations from my memories of them. To protect privacy, in some instances I have changed the names of individuals and places, I may have changed some identifying characteristics and details such as physical properties, occupations and places of residence.

www.newgeneration-publishing.com

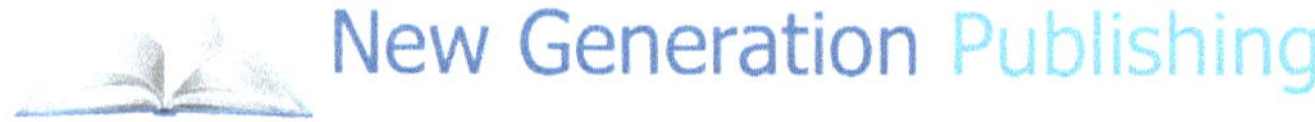

ABOUT THE AUTHOR

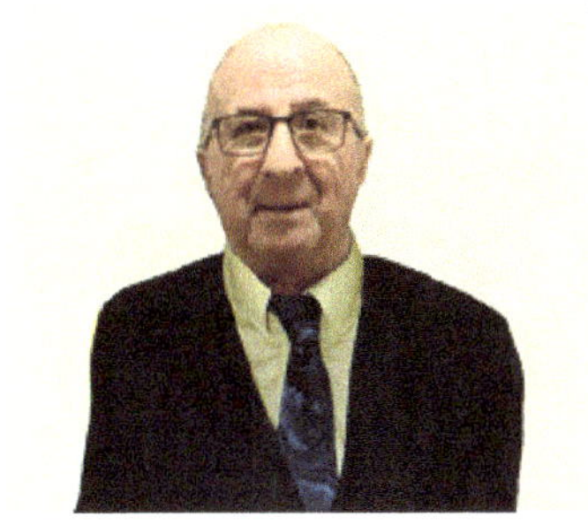

This book reveals the struggles that Michael experienced throughout his life, including the doctors telling his parents that he would never read and write.

In his teenage years, he was unable to relate properly to members of the opposite sex. He often felt left out and very upset seeing them with boyfriends.

It wasn't until later in life that Michael started to behave like other people in his own age group. He went on to gain qualifications in City and Guilds in Painting and Decorating and others besides.

Since then, Michael has developed and has a good life, living independently on his own in sheltered accommodation.

Despite his disability, he has made and continues to make considerable effort to communicate and stay in touch with a wide variety of friends and family.

INTRODUCTION

One day in 1997, my mother saw one of many television programs on autistic spectrum disorders. She wished to know more about the condition and what she had heard so far fitted my criteria and simultaneously a conference was taking place at the Maudsley Hospital, South London on Autistic Spectrum Condition (ASC.)

Rather than miss out, I thought of this as a great opportunity attending; when told about the conference, I made my mind up by supporting the event and so, one sunny cold October morning, I started making my way there.

On arrival I met others with the same condition or similar. It saw a new Chapter in life getting to know many contacts over time. Including one patient I knew previously at the Maudsley and catching up with him many years later.

Through attending the conference, it opened up many avenues and in the spring of 1998 I was already finding out whether I had autism and undergoing many tests including an IQ test and brain scan.

Throughout my life, I have always known that I was different but I did not know what was wrong. I have found things hard, very frustrating and painful. My life has been blighted and my mental and physical health have both been affected. "Where was the help I needed throughout most of my life"? I have been fending for myself so far but having this diagnosis has opened some doors of support for me and has helped me understand myself better.

I have been lucky in that I had a loyal, loving and supportive mother until her demise in 2015 and currently I have two sisters and an extended family and social network supporting me. I have lived an independent life since the age of 25 including: shopping, cooking, cleaning, handling my finances and I am computer literate.

My disability is most distinct when it comes to relating and communicating with other people. In this respect I continue to struggle and I am longing for a feeling of a sense of connection and companionship, belonging and finding a place in the community and feeling accepted and one day finding somebody who understands my needs so that I may settle down with that one special person.

Throughout my life, I found things hard, very frustrating and painful. All through having autism and hardly understood until at least, my late 40's.

Michael Feldman

CHAPTER ONE

EARLY YEARS

1. Early Signs Of Autism

My life began in East London in 1950 in two bedrooms of a shared house. On the first floor was our family consisting of my parents, my older sister, and me. We lived in a friendly neighbourhood and it felt that autism wasn't a problem as I was getting along well with my neighbours.

Before I was born my mother thought that I was a little late moving in the womb. So she saw her doctor about the flutter absence. She must have been at least twenty weeks into her pregnancy when the problem started. Theoretically this is the most exciting time when a mother should feel the baby kicking inside her.

I was born two weeks later than average and my mother always said that I had a normal birth and development until having whooping cough at around three months old. I was admitted to hospital and whilst I was getting over whooping cough I contracted pneumonia and then gastroenteritis followed. I survived these conditions but then contracted Chicken Pox at nine months.

When I started recovering from these illnesses, my mother started to notice that my development may have been delayed. Whether this was related to the illnesses or I was born with my condition will always be unknown. I was unable to sit up without support until eleven months old and my physical mobility was delayed considerably. At twenty-two months, I started taking my first steps. Usually babies learn to walk much earlier than this.

In these early years my parents noticed that I was not behaving in the way that my sister had at the same age. I was often rocking in my chair which continued until five years of age.

At age two or two and a half I started to make noises and my first attempt at speech was at age three and a half. I was linking only small sentences together and I was constantly repeating what others were saying. My conversation consisted of asking loads of questions with one or two statements until I was about eleven or twelve years of age.

My mother often said that in these early days she felt as if she were a walking encyclopaedia, answering whatever questions I threw at her. I was constantly frustrated and wanted to know the answers to the same questions over and over again. An example would be "What went pop?" with the same expected answer being.." A balloon".

Throughout my childhood my parents had to deal with a range of frustrations that were often irrational for example if a toy car fell on the floor I would cry for hours on end over this trivial incident.

Things hardly changed outside. One day I was taken to a newsagent shop where I urinated up against the counter. To the shopkeeper's displeasure, he came out with a facetious remark "It's the morning papers that you have been reading".

Finding this far from funny my mother could have taken action against the shop keeper resulting in giving him a right pasting. With such ignorance he felt unable to make allowances for anyone with an impairment.

So at this time of my life I felt unable to control

my emotions and had little or no social skills. At eight years of age I was getting upset for no reason including misinterpreting what my family were saying and crying and wailing over and over in the process......

"WHAT DID YOU SAYYYYYY!!?"
"WHAT DID YOU SAYYYYYY!!?"

My father, whatever he said, was failing to register that sometimes whatever is said can be misinterpreted. So, with poor language and developmental skills you can see how frustrating life was for all of us and this was not all.

2. Out Of The Ordinary

Many autistic children at a young age are unaware of danger. I was far from immune and wish to share this incident and others taking place throughout my childhood

One hot summer's day, my family decided to go to Southend for the day. When we arrived the beach was very crowded with many families deciding to take advantage of the good weather and also getting away from the pressures of work and enjoying any time they had.

My parents too must have had the same idea and oblivious on what was to happen next, started setting up space. As they were settling down, I started observing a group of swimmers taking turns jumping off a nearby jetty and with no common sense and taking into account that I couldn't swim I decided in joining them.

My parents and Norma clearly saw that I was running towards the swimmers. She yelled hoping that I would stop. I carried on getting as far as where they were jumping and appearing to be ignoring Norma's plea before getting to the end of the jetty. Jumping in and going beneath the surface.

Almost immediately I heard gurgling noises similar to a bottle submerged in water and bubbles rising to the surface and going deeper and deeper and swallowing water at various intervals.

With Norma shouting frantically waving her arms a swimmer saw her and with no hesitation jumping in and catching sight, took hold before making his way to the surface, to my family's relief.

Feeling the least scared, Norma, saw that surprised look on my face on going under and resurfacing. I must have 'blacked out' by the time a swimmer came to my aid and started pulling me from the murky depths.

In between I remembered nothing else until regaining consciousness at the top of the jetty.

As a rough guess, many onlookers on shore were watching the drama unfold with at least 20 or 30 swimmers present that day. So with the worst happening and that I wasn't "coming back"' that I shudder thinking of the dreadful consequences with my family, returning from Southend to an empty house with one less family member.

Soon and subsequently "coming too" my mother appeared on the scene. Thanking the person responsible for saving my life. Following things through she firmly took hold and rushed back along the jetty to where we were settling down and trying to make use of the time left.

This act alone was so foolish and having no swimming experience to show for that I was failing to pick up on the dangers and making out to my parents how unaware that the water was that deep.

So far and with events unfolding that day and about a week or so following the incident I thought about going back to Southend. Leading up to this my father was delivering leaflets at a nearby council estate. It had a fair sized hall, a childrens' play area and a local church nearby.

By the time he started deviating elsewhere I parted company. Making my way to the high road and catching a bus to get to Fenchurch Street Station in East London. Even at my age, and knowing that one could get to Southend from there, that I was eventually seen by the bus conductor and told to get off at Hackney Police Station.

Soon discovering my disappearance my father took another bus and succeeded by catching up and retorting, "You mustn't run away like that" before handing me an apple and thinking that I was happy as we were prepared to go home.

As usual, my parents continued taking us to Southend or Chalkwell. This time, I brought a crab home and left a bucket near the stairs with the crab inside, little knowing that the crab was bound to escape. So, unaware of it creeping out by hearing the slightest of scuttling, it started making its way down towards my neighbour living beneath.

At first thought my downstairs neighbour, Lily, thought it was a tarantula spider and she got the fright of her life and screaming in terror. So far and until this period this incident was bad enough until worse was to come and, having a conscience for the first time.

One night I was playing in the bathroom splashing water all over the place and unaware of it making its way through the floorboards and into my neighbour's living room. Unaware of the fate coming next the damage had already been done with water flowing steadily through the ceiling. In the process, my neighbours tried preventing as much damage to the carpets as possible by catching the water in a bucket; within a few minutes and witnessing the event unfolding, the flow reduced to a trickle before stopping completely.

Making my way upstairs Norma saw that I was upset and asking me to stop crying. So, it appeared that I was having some feeling towards other people; I thought too, that through acting foolishly, my downstairs neighbours may have known about my condition and feeling inclined asking my parents to pay for the damage.

When things were back to normal I continued acting

silly and more than any normal 5 year old when 'The Westminster Waltz' was played on the radio in the mid to late 1950's. It seemed a popular choice for anyone into the mellow side of music.

By coincidence the tune happened to be around as Bonfire Night was getting when Norma decided to make a guy. Stuffing a pillowcase full of clothing and a yellow mask to complete the finishing touches and placing the guy on the armchair.

Unaware of the guy's presence, I accidentally sat on top of it, damaging the mask in the process. Since this instance I found myself acting odd, eccentric or silly and singing, 'oh the guy's a sheer' each time the tune appeared on the radio.'

Norma and my parents, found it funny and ever since, things are still elusive in how I came to singing those ridiculous lyrics. At this time, I was having some mischievous and happy moments taking place between the lulls in between misbehaving.

When things were bad I was often upsetting Norma and recalling many years later in a subdued moment that I was, over this period, failing to be like "normal" brothers. She also knew about my challenging behaviour and pulling her hair and perhaps, made allowances given the fact of my untoward behaviour.

Also in the times that followed, Norma and I enjoyed jumping off the wardrobe. Landing on our beds in the process and almost definitely, weakening the springs in the process. Through my condition and what appeared fun at any rate, I also enjoyed........

Throwing spoons down the toilet
Throwing pots brooms and pans down the stairs

These last two episodes of mischief, included part of the fun with an unknown theory....

"Was my hyperactivity down to what I ate? In the 1950's, many foods had additives causing hyperactivity."

"Was it down to 'coming out of my shell' and showing off or, whether I knew what I was doing and simultaneously unaware of the noise from these items coming down the stairs.

By my parents knowing any answers, I felt, would at least be getting to the route of my problems. That is the issue of certain foods making children hyperactive and only known many years later. This in general, is what one should focus on coupled with the many guidelines available online in dealing with hyperactive children.

Generalising these points, many children enjoy getting up to mischievous things and sometimes, excited too over little things.

At 5 years of age I was clearly showing my excitement by my parents purchasing a television; including perfect strangers; reciting ....

"WE'VE GOT A TELEVISION!"

With my excitement clearly 'rubbing off' on onlookers on a shopping trip, that they may have made some allowances for this as I was already in a push chair. So for many onlookers (or perfect strangers) they may have thought that I was younger than my 5 years.

My family however could see the excitement clearly written all over my face. For many televisions were very pricey and owning one around the mid 1950's was a luxury for the privileged few.

This was the norm until the early to mid 1950's and before, with excited children seeing a neighbour bringing back a car and running out of their front doors to greet the driver; in this specific period many people were so poor, that some of them had to count every penny before buying the necessary essentials.

In the late 1950's, more householders could afford a

television. Including my family and downstairs neighbours and perceived as a novelty at first.

Very soon, and with my excitement diminishing, my parents saw that I was getting upset through missing the beginning of a particular programme and, resulting with my reluctance seeing the programme through to the end. So, a family member tried pretending to get the programme to start from the beginning. I soon however got wise to his ploy and once more was reluctant watching what was left of the programme. This was the way I was as well as episodes of hyperactivity and an Associated Learning Difference and formerly called A Learning Difficulty.

On top of the issues I was having I also had trouble trying to have control over myself and apparent when starting school and hardly mixing with anyone.

3. The Assessment

In the early or middle part of the 1950's I was to undergo one of many assessments since little was known about autism until it's discovery in 1943.

On the day of the appointment taking place, my parents explained to the doctor about my bizarre behaviour of kissing everyone on the head, including the doctor's. I did exactly that by entering his room and kissing his head in the process. Immediately, he may have been taken aback and brushing aside things and failing to comment.

One very good reason for his reaction was seeing children with similar behaviour many times before. So, giving an account and a general picture of how I was, he decided that I should see a psychologist. Things however were made clear that I was failing in making little progress.

This time, the psychologist thought that with an IQ of only 50 that he knew the possibility of a good education was poor, as throughout much of the assessment I was acting up on the tests.

To my parents, things went beyond a joke when the psychologist retorted "Put the spoon in the cup"; disobeying his command I ended up throwing the spoon about or hitting the spoon still in the cup that it would fall to the floor breaking into little pieces.

By keeping my hyperactivity under control and with the right medication I also felt that I could have acted more normally and obtaining better results in the process.

With a low IQ and an ongoing condition the psychologist felt about Fountain Hospital in Tooting, South London. An institution for handicapped children with the reality of 600 children attending in an overcrowded environment.

All of this was in the 1950's and a coinciding waiting list for 170 patients was already in play; the beds were so far together that it felt very cumbersome moving around.

The huts too were temporary, dilapidated and run-down; the barrack or comparable wards in these huts had no recreation room; so the children were unable to play in bad weather.

With a second doctor intervening on my parents' behalf, I was spared from any 'first hand' experience at this hospital.

At the Consultation my parents could have done without the doctor's negative comments that I would never read and write. His outspoken comments were upsetting both of them. In the end, these turned out false and I got to 'shine' when it came to reading and showing at residential school.

The remarkable qualities pertaining to my reading came with a reading age of 10 and by coincidence, at 10 years of age. This was seen as an achievement; I had the highest reading age among my classroom peers; so, something to be proud of by any standard with the professionals stating that I would never read or write along with ending up as an uncontrollable adult.

Unsurprisingly, hearing these negative comments

both my parents were on the verge of seeking a second opinion. The doctors at County Hall knew of a Harley Street Neurologist, a Dr WD. One of the many doctors practising in this well-known street consisting of various professionals ranging from dentists, opticians, general practitioners and so on.

My parents were so desperate, that they were only too pleased getting the referral from County Hall. With caring parents, they had my wellbeing to heart or, so that I could at least act normal and act the same as other children.

Eagerly waiting for the appointment, I was seen by a Dr WD who thought of me as severely abnormal and prescribing Phenobarbitone or Etherdrine to slow me down and glutamic acid for stimulating my brain for making one less hyperactive.

At the next appointment he arranged a follow-up IQ test with one of his psychologists. This time increasing to 73.

To my parents' relief the tests were favourable and that I was subsequently capable in receiving a good education. At this consultation a second doctor had me on her lap and repeating the previous task accomplished at County Hall and asserting abruptly. **"PUT THE SPOON IN THE CUP!"** This time her efforts worked resulting in an improvement with my performance. However, continuing unaware what I was letting myself in for at Dr WD's surgery, where I found myself playing around with his dog, a Yorkshire Terrier and failing to realise that the dog had the desire to be left alone. I refused picking up on this and ended up getting bitten on the hand.

Whatever problems I had my mother was under so much stress and exhaustion that she had a nervous breakdown. At a young age I was unable to help the way I was in between her recovery in hospital and my family who were temporarily separated.

Norma, my sister, was staying with grandparents in

Edgware, Middlesex. I was staying with my grandparents on my mother's side; the location was Stoke Newington, North London and lasting until her recovery where we resumed as a normal family.

About this time, or a year or so later I was attending a kindergarten called Fernbank.

At the kindergarten, the staff knew the meaning of the word, 'disabled' and more than I can say when some parents collecting their children were unforthcoming, making insulting remarks saying.. "Put him in a home, he's mad."

These people may have contributed to my mother's anxiety or she may have coped and avoid going to hospital.

Whatever the reasons with my mischievous behaviour, their remark "Put him in a home" was down to plain ignorance.

At kindergarten, I remember running into the nursery's kitchen for amusement as one of the mischievous acts that I was capable of at 3 to 4 years of age.

When things did get better in the last days of kindergarten and at almost 5 years of age, I was taken to Clarke's College. A private institute in East London. For the occasion, my mother purchased a uniform.

When we arrived we were introduced to the principle and I was placed in a class with children of my age all alone in this strange environment. My mother made her way to my grandparents. A 15 minute bus ride away. She was only there for four hours when she received a phone call from the college about my intolerant behaviour and through acting up and interrupting the lessons I had to go; sadly, my brand-new uniform was a waste of money.

All what was left now, was to see out the last few months at Kindergarten and starting mainstream school in East London. The year is 1956.

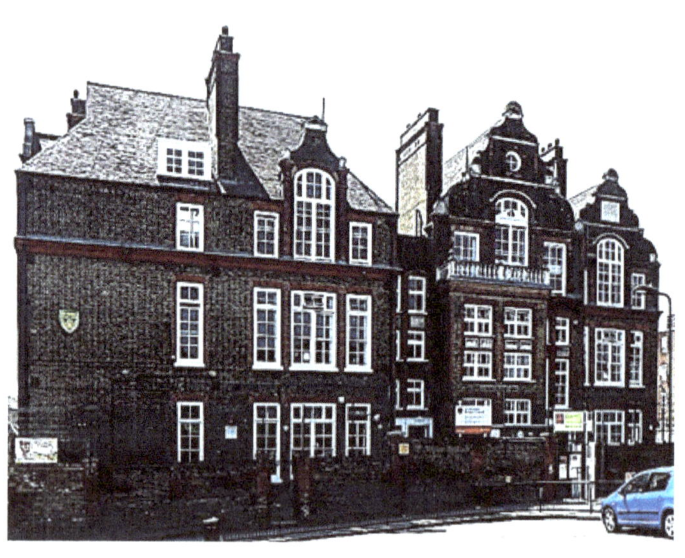

My first School, Southwold.

CHAPTER TWO

FIRST SCHOOL

1. Happiest Years

The nearest school to where we lived was Southwold. It was mainstream with my first day beginning around 6th January 1956. This was a start preparing for the outside world by developing a decent education and starting employment or advancing to college or university.

Over the coming days, I found myself settling down, and conforming to this new beginning.

In the same year I secured a friendship with a classmate, John, a very pleasant 'chap' along with my teacher with the requisites by making many individuals happy.

My family was often inviting him round to my house and I now believe that the reality developing a life time friendship was there. Both of us were 5 years of age and enjoyed having fun; for a laugh, playing hide and seek. My job was trying to find John and coming across him hiding in a cupboard.

As my first real friend and lasting for a very long time, that I can see this as a real achievement, or I may have had more friends falling back on from kindergarten. So far I had adequate social skills or sense of direction and arising when sent to the local delicatessen for ½lb of butter and sugar.

The ironic thing at only five years of age that my family seemed confident enough with my ability to shop alone without getting lost. They had no worries with my safe arrival back home.

Today however is a 'far cry' from that as many parents are afraid of letting their children perform these errands. Finding this pathetic, kids can no longer roam around safely through the risk of falling into the hands of low-life 'scum bags.' When I was growing up nobody had any worries and felt lucky going out on our own and happily playing in our local neighbourhood.

Helping things further our teacher, was seen as a very kind lady and very good friends with my mother, many years later. Everybody was fond of her including other pupils and staff too were seeing her as very kind and able to have a good conversation with.

She was also a fine pianist and resulting in us always looking forward to her music sessions. Singing along to the tunes of the day and clearly enjoying ourselves.

Since settling in at school, the happiest years of my life were between 1956 and 1959. I appeared to be settling down and conforming with everyone, things were appearing as a 'step in the right direction.'

Wishing that this trend were to continue, may have seen my happiest years extended over a certain period; by 1959, things were about to change with my challenging behaviour and driving the teachers to distraction and, simultaneously, getting smacked.

2 Acting Incompatibly

By the time of reaching 8 years of age, I was getting up to much mischief; away from my present teacher. I was in another class where the teacher in charge was drawing attention in front of everyone that she would smack my backside and adding. "Do you know what your backside is?" I replied "No." She replied, "It's your bottom."

With so much ignorance around carrying out the appropriate punishments was allowed in schools and institutions.

According to my family, I was often driving the teachers to tears. They knew that I was a tearaway and failing to learn a great deal. I hardly tried interacting with my peers and choosing to be alone most times.

In the break periods and on many an occasion, I had fun taking sheets of toilet paper and throwing them up in the air in windy weather. This was my act of fun until a teacher started having other thoughts. Interjecting that the sheets of paper were contributing to a litter problem and that nobody else was acting this way; perhaps making paper planes and seeing them fly, may have been the better and sensible option.

Norma, my sister, in the Juniors section knew about my mischievous behaviour and found herself often speaking to my teacher. Losing or throwing away my dinner money, was no exception. I was wrapping the money in paper and throwing away the contents outside a block of flats and thinking no more of my actions.

At lunch time the teachers were helping where they could and waiving the fact that I had no money available and giving me free lunch; sometimes after lunch, I often enjoyed walking to Millfields Park in East London and comprising of four playing fields with overlooking flats and houses and a children's play area.

The park was only 5 minutes away from our school with a fair number of children seen in fine weather. Including an older pupil Henry, was no exception. He had blonde hair, appeared friendly and, tall for his age. On this fine, sunny day I saw him leisurely paddling near the children's play area and offering a piggy back in the process. Suddenly, I unsuccessfully tried holding on to him until landing in the pool and getting soaked to the skin.

As the break ended I had no other clothes to change into until my teacher, handed a replacement. Right from the start, I felt unhappy changing into a fresh set of clothing with the nearest laundrette a mile or so away. It seemed an impossible task getting them dry in time for afternoon lessons or when it was time to go home.

When it was time to go home I entered a neighbour's garden and changed back into the soaking wet clothes that I already had and leaving the dry ones behind. At school the next day I heard nothing more.

As a loner and virtually failing to make new friends I was on the odd occasion failing to return in time for lessons. Nearby were some of the 'older form,' about to make their way back to school.

Choosing to stay obstinate and reluctant by returning to school, I chose on roaming around Millfields until one day I was dragged back to my class by these lads. On the way, I continued 'throwing tantrums' through failure in getting my own way.

At least the 4 lads involved appeared friendly enough. I can now perceive them as acting appropriately by ensuring my safe arrival and joining my fellow 'class mates.' In this period too almost everybody had much admiration with no teasing or making fun.

The nearest anyone got by any teasing came with two compares playing a light-hearted joke when a Punch and Judy Show was taking place.

With the show in full swing the compares of the show were unable to take off Mr Punch how he usually speaks and making do with their natural voices.

As a joke one of them ended up saying. "Michael is a nut case." Calling out back, I retorted, "Don't you talk to me like that!" Both kids I thought meant no offence and have to say that I have no hard feelings towards them.

My aim is trying to avoid unpleasant situations, keeping out of trouble and keeping within the boundaries;

knowing how far I can go with certain people before they themselves end up rude or plain discourteous.

Back in 1959, things were a far cry when at 8 years of age I continued throwing tantrums and bringing myself to the attention of perfect strangers. This was part of my autism and happened one hot summer's day when taken to Millfields Park.

With the warm weather already upon us I decided on wearing a coat and reluctant to take it off, I ended up causing a scene. Crying out loud and throwing a tantrum in front of onlookers ignoring my pleas and perhaps, seeing that I was naughty.

By gradually calming down my family succeeded in taking off my coat. With the tantrums that I was having, they were sort of an everyday occurrence. I was often unaware of my social surroundings with one of many classic examples arising one summer's evening at Springfield Park.

One evening I came across a game of bowls taking place in the distance and should have been watching the game in play. Having second thoughts, I thought of intruding onto the bowling green and refusing to leave when told to do so.

As a family member was already in the park he heard from a distance a disturbance taking place. With no hesitation he could see that I was acting up, took hold and dragged me all the way back home. I started throwing another one of my tantrums with the local neighbours looking on from the flats opposite the park.

The players involved in the bowling incident were middle-aged and unaware of my impairment, may have put things down to disobedience before getting back to their game.

My behaviour already was challenging and mischievous too in school and in the community. At school, I made everyone laugh by performing in my teacher's, absence. Performing a head stand on her chair and making the whole class laugh hysterically, making myself the centre of attention.

I often made many of my peers very happy with how I behaved. Now everybody was thinking that I was eccentric by playing with my teacher's hair; saying out aloud for everyone to hear. "Let me fiddle with your hair!"

My classmates observing my strange behaviour, were brushing things aside or I may have been labelled as 'weirdo' or 'Spastic', words often used in my earlier years and beyond.

The mentality to any civilised person was no way forward, going about 'calling names' to anyone with behaviour problems; autism is one of many disabilities blighting or ruining many lives. Including **my own** and making my presence felt further.

Any one knowing the meaning of **autism** will see it as no picnic with most individuals met with sheer frustrations and for some, feeling very disturbed, seeing themselves getting into trouble. Even today, I am still not immune.

In the course of my life many peers or associates may have taken me at 'face value' or accepting who I was.

One good thing about my popularity, seeing the opportunity clearly, thereby making further friends when one kid, out of the goodness of his heart gave me a quantity of dinky toys. A craze going around was...Lining up two dinkies side by side and using marbles for each opponent to aim at the toys. When hitting the toys, the lucky opponent gets to keep them.

We definitively had something in common; by any friendship developing I could begin seeing him outside at any of the play centres, giving children somewhere to play; the play centres always existed in the holidays where I often attended.

At one of the centres, I continue recalling a funny incident taking place in the play area.

Nearby to where I stood, a kid was filling up a metal

water tray with water and consisting of sand, a bucket and spade and a rubber funnel. As he pressed the funnel flat water started to spurt out of it and I fell into hysterics with laughter until it started hindering my breathing.

When I calmed down I carried on as normal. I was the only one laughing so much and compared to laughing softly or something better to laugh about.

By attending the play centres a slight improvement showed in my behaviour. The staff were reporting back to my parents less often except with faltering behaviour.

In between periods I continued getting up to no good trying to dig up a birdhouse situated alongside a block of flats. In the process two kids nearby were advising that I should stop.

With the weight of it being too heavy trying to take it home, their advice was very sensible; one of kids however, appeared to have a strange look about him and looked the 'criminal' type.

As the new term began a teacher arranged a tape recording session and compared with the 'funnel' incident, this was far from funny. When my turn came to say something, I accused one of the kids in the 'bird house incident,' a thief. I was coming out with the most ridiculous remark "He's a burglar", trying to 'tarnish' his reputation.

Things were appearing that I had real social issues and my remark could have seen my popularity plummeting among my fellow peers; my life too may have been too uncomfortable to the point in leaving primary school altogether. I was often getting on the wrong side of people including observing a group of builders working on the school surroundings and getting into trouble with them.

I felt unaware of my conduct when visiting their hut in breaks. So I was seen as an unwelcome pest and failing to pick up on this. At first they thought little of my behaviour, until constantly knocking on the shed door until told to "scarper" or depart suddenly.

Still failing to listen, a member from the team opened

the door and without hesitation, started hitting me around the head. So, learning things the hard way, I stopped pestering them further.

My parents however may have taken a different view with them taking this individual to court; neither my parents or the school knew about this incident. The culprit responsible for his actions saw the opportunity reporting any wrong doing to the teachers.

Throughout my time the teachers were the only ones carrying out some form of corporal punishment until one kid and for some unknown reason took a disliking to me through my autism or through the way I behaved.

Making my way home one day I met up with him and for no apparent reason, I got hit in the head and stomach and left alone to recover; this lad looked the rough type or, plain cowardice on his part for targeting the weaker or vulnerable type.

With his wrongdoing I tried getting even with him. Hitting him without any success and ending as a farce; I wasn't hurting him enough and meeting him again, his words were.... "Now you gave me a few, so I shall give you a couple" before backing off with no further instances arising.

In the late 50's and to the present day school bullying continues existing and that most kids report their wrongdoing counterparts to a staff member. I failed on this and felt that I should have been thankful that the 'run-ins' that I had with this kid, didn't last long.

At 8 years of age, occasionally my father and my mother tapped me as a form of smacking. I was lacking any judgement and when coming across a police officer I asked him to '*put my Mum and Dad in prison.*'

In utter amazement, he started asking 'Why?' I replied '*Mummy and Daddy keep on smacking me.*" Still amazed and wondering what to make of things, he saw that I wasn't distressed, or injured and decided that no further action was needed.

I may have been too young to be charged for any offence and found myself in a spot of trouble when failing to return home from school one day. At the spur of the moment I took a leisurely stroll along Lea Bridge Road and started running along Millfields. With my fellow peers absent to intervene as before when overstaying my time in the park I took the opportunity of going further afield.

Heading towards the entrance to Hackney Marshes a police officer came into view. He must have known about my parent's anxiety when receiving a call on his radio about my absence from home.

As he caught up he stopped and started making some enquiries before taking hold and advancing to a police kiosk for the purpose of calling one of his officers. Back in the day they served a purpose for calling and reporting a crime taking place.

Under the given circumstances and with my parents worried sick, that he could have at least saved 5 minutes by using his radio in comparison to visiting the kiosk. When we got there, he called for his colleague before being taken home and reunited with my family.

On the way home I perceived him as coming across as friendly and easy to talk to; as we got to my home, his friendliness vanished; changing his tune, I could clearly see that authoritarian look on him and looking extremely unpleasant.

The most shameful thing came about each time I failed looking at him, he would shout aloud.....

"LOOK AT ME!!"

For an 8 year old this can be so intimidating for any child and beyond belief. I am thinking to myself...

"How could this officer get away with such uncalled for behaviour?"

In passing conversation I clearly saw him angry

about my absence and about the worry on my mother's face especially. In my view he was **certainly** getting his point across in a nasty way compared to acting more professional about my absence from home.

In my early years or at the time of this incident happening ignorance against disabled people was prevalent or widespread in the 1950's; 'on the surface,' most autistics look the same as anyone else.

The policeman had no idea about the meaning of autism and had no empathy. Some autistic people also find it hard **LOOKING** directly at people. This meant nothing to him, or I could see him showing more respect by finding out the reasons for failing to come home and most importantly warning me of the dangers of certain undesirables around and taking it upon themselves by harming a child physically or sexually.

With the lack of understanding I felt in addition in dealing with the matter he could have been more professional by showing patience and tolerance by **ABSTAINING** from insisting on direct eye contact, speaking very clearly and evaluating the type of mood that I might have been in at the time and better than frightening anyone at a very young age. Adding too, the ignorance by shouting and undermining anyone is totally inappropriate and unacceptable.

To the relief of my sister, Norma and my parents, a brief respite came in my abnormal behaviour when I learned to ride a two wheeler bicycle.

Until now, I continued riding a three wheeler until getting on for 9 years of age. Things were about to change when our next door neighbours had a son. He owned a two-wheeler bicycle and was keen on lending it to out for practice. Until requesting it back.

Following his request I flatly refused and resulting in a choice by informing his parents or my family about my behaviour. He chose my father and as he came down the stairs and into the street I was dragged off his bike and taken upstairs to my bedroom.

In the process of taking off my clothes I was throwing one of my usual tantrums and trying to get away from him. I failed and finally setting out his intentions by putting me to bed and locking the door behind him; I was refusing to accept that what I did was wrong by my refusal by handing his bike back.

Almost immediately and with an escape plan in mind I lowered myself out the bedroom window and landed on a roof about 10 feet down; my next course of action was to lower myself over a garden wall, walk round to the street where we lived and get the bike off him.

Nearby were my clothes and I made it down as far as my neighbour's garden when they started catching sight and calling for my father to intervene. By grabbing hold for a second time, I tried getting away as he was making his way to my room and in the process and in a 'sulky' manner, I was saying. "I want to have a practice!!"

This meant very little to him other than jokingly, saying "I'll practice on your bottom" knowing full well that I wanted to get back on his bike. It wasn't going to happen! Through my episodes of wrongdoing he took off my clothes, and gently smacked my bare backside for every item of clothing I had on me.."One for the trousers!." "one for the shirt!" and so on and having my clothes taken away and returned the following morning.

On most occasions when chastised by my parents I usually failed listening to reason with one exception ie acting more reasonably towards him when 'calling time' or meeting his request by returning his bike.

By co-operating this time round I learnt to ride his two wheeler bicycle in 5 days. By the time I was almost 11½ years of age in 1962 we were very good friends; I was more settled emotionally in comparison with my in-patient stay at the Maudsley Hospital between 1959 to 1961.

In this present period I was continually disturbed and disruptive.

My work performance was poor, I was often smacked by the teachers with my own teacher on one occasion pulling my pants down and smacking my bare backside with a slipper. By trying to correct my behaviour using this method, also saw them failing unsuccessfully.

Today any teacher performing this way would mean instant dismissal and putting his/her chances of teaching in jeopardy. During my childhood corporal punishment was a form of correction with many children thinking twice about telling their parents through fear of getting smacked themselves.

3. Last Attempt

At other people's expense, I continued getting into trouble, including in the Jewish Community. So, with no exception, I saw a Jewish kid walking along my road and attempted to steal his hat; in real terms and in the Jewish religion, the hat is a 'kippah'.

As he was trying to pass I tried taking it off him when, almost immediately, I was pushed so hard that my head hit the pavement. With little harm done, I made my way home as if nothing had happened, with a second act of foolishness coming soon after. I was at a nearby synagogue and, intentionally, entered a class where a Hebrew lesson was taking place. With no courtesy, I opened the classroom door and immediately, my words were, "I'm coming to Hebrew."

Suddenly, the teacher stopped the lesson with his pupils thinking it odd seeing somebody with my character, acting 'out of the ordinary'. By failing to take my impairment into account, he thought that I was messing around and took action by showing me into a room looking similar to a prison cell and locked the door.

Opposite was a window wide enough to successfully escape through by climbing onto a table and, inconspicuously, leaving the Schul [synagogue] without being seen – until deciding to try the same thing again. This time in passing, I was told, "Do you remember when I locked you up?" "Yes, but I managed to get away."

Realising that I had an impairment, I was allowed to leave the synagogue; so taking no further action the second time round, I stopped interrupting his lessons altogether. On both occasions, I failed by telling my parents about my ordeal.

Since this experience, I heard many years later that he had a reputation of locking misbehaved pupils in cupboards. Sometimes, his wrongdoings caught up with him and I'm recalling one incident by hearsay – a parent of one pupil hit him so hard that he fell to the ground.

By informing my parents what happened, the police may have been involved and he may have 'done time' in prison. In this period and beyond, I'm saying to myself…

"**HOW COULD HE** sink that low, holding prisoner anyone daring to misbehave in his presence and locking them up in the process? Anyone under his care may have also been having doubts about his position of teaching in the first place."

Believing that this individual should be put to shame, that he was 'falling down' by handling things better and advising on knocking first and in an appropriate manner, asking…

"Can I help in any way?"

"I would like to join your Hebrew class" would have been my reply.

Appropriately answering my request, he may have advised by enrolling, or, speaking to the principal for further advice in joining.

By recalling this incident, I felt that I was completely unaware of my conduct and upsetting his class on impulse. I felt that I was unable to control my actions and that many more incidents were to follow. Including my next act of foolishness.

One day, I spotted an owner cleaning his car. By his side, he had car shampoo and a bucket of water on the other. Seeing the opportunity, I deliberately kicked the bucket hard enough for the contents to spill into the road. I felt lucky however that the guy was 'easy going' and avoiding any confrontation taking place.

This was the beginning of 'acting up' whenever I could. Another incident arose by knocking a tin of paint off a step ladder; the resident at the time was painting a wall outside his front door. So, jumping to the opportunity, I crossed the road and knocked the tin of paint off the step ladder; immediately I found myself 'held prisoner' and taken into his house before I started to cry. His intentions were to call the police, until I was pleading and begging for him to let me go.

With common sense and against calling the police, he saved himself facing a kidnap charge and prison to follow. When I was finally allowed to go, I uttered a few choice words before disappearing quietly off the scene and leaving him to clear up the mess. So, learning my lesson the 'hard way' I felt deterred from any further incidents of this kind, of getting into trouble outside of school.

School was just as bad with continuing poor education and I was getting up to further mischief as before. With poor education, my prospects of getting a reasonable job later in life must have been virtually non-existent, or, settling for dead-end positions – jobs consisting of poor pay.

My parents tried other avenues. They arrived at private tuition. The first teacher (or tutor) was a middle-aged man with mousy hair. My parents, thinking that I wasn't getting very far with this tutor, decided on finding another tutor and, hoping that he could get my education to an acceptable standard, this was soon arranged. In the beginning, I went with Norma to his house until becoming familiar with directions, then seeing myself through making my way there on my own.

As I got to his house, he appeared mild mannered and showed some compassion on one of my visits when I was in tears because the satchel that I was carrying came away because of a broken strap. At the time, I was already having private tuition as in copying one exercise, italic writing exercises consisting of joined letters in this sentence as one given example…

Zoe quickly mixed up the seven big jars of sweets.

Over time, the exercises would gradually improve. Learning to write as neatly as possible in comparison to writing untidily.

I felt that with the right tuition the chances were there, seeing my education improving much sooner than later and simultaneously feeling calm and, finally, the 'icing on the cake' – the possibility of continuing my education at Southwold and advancing to senior, or grammar school by passing the 11 plus.

Despite trying his best to improve my education, he was unsuccessful. So my parents had to try elsewhere to get my education to an executable standard and, to achieve this, it was going to take much time.

So with the mischief that I was getting up to, I had no friends at all. Also more disappointment came with an open day taking place at Southwold back in 1959 and seeing many parents supporting it. Mr The Headmaster had no choice but filling in my family that I was hardly learning.

I was at or around nine years of age and so hyperactive. The Head also added that I was the most impaired child that he had ever come across; the 'autism subject' was avoided throughout narrating his piece; in its place he may have been thinking on the terms of attending a suitable institution where I could at least, start obtaining a better education. When saying this, it could have been with good intentions, thinking that I would fare better elsewhere.

His suggestions were upsetting my parents greatly and so, and thinking to myself…

"Now who can my parents turn to?"

"At the age of nine years and knowing no better about changing my circumstances, what else could I do?"

"Would I have fared any better elsewhere, as The Headmaster expressed with interest in passing and was trying to mean well?"

Answering my own question:

"Yes." On the proviso of any special schools or institutes existing in the area. With the exception and, as far as knowing, none existed for ASCs (Autistic Spectrum Conditions) and/or for the ESN (Educationally Sub Normal) or a more subtle phrase, a Specific Learning Difference.

With the lack of resources available in 1959, my parents soon heard from their local GP of Maudsley Hospital in South London and I'm guessing that they were thinking to themselves…

"Was there going to be a 'chink' of light at the end of the tunnel and earning the break they needed with my problems?"

As a good choice, things appeared to be turning out well, with Maudsley at this time the better option; it was a residential hospital for disturbed children and those with behavioural and/or specific learning differences.

I met this criteria and it was to be a start for staff members helping to turn my life around and a 'stepping stone' platform before starting boarding school under a two-year timescale.

At the time of leaving Southwold, I was still hyperactive and coinciding with this period the doctors assumed I had psychosis or, *a severe mental disorder in which thought and impaired emotions is tantamount (or equal) to lost contact and external reality.*

Their assumptions may have been an exaggeration, and better described as a behavioural disorder as more the norm. So, with my final presence at Southwold one morning, my Southwold associates were to gradually realise that I was no longer at school and, in the process, were feeling very upset; I was admired by many, generalising the 'bigger picture'. I find it ironic that my impairment was no barrier to having popularity periods.

Also, it was sad for Norma, feeling that as the brother that she was hoping for was absent from her life. I saw her constantly putting up with my erratic and eccentric behaviour. Now feeling very sad, she was about to miss me terribly.

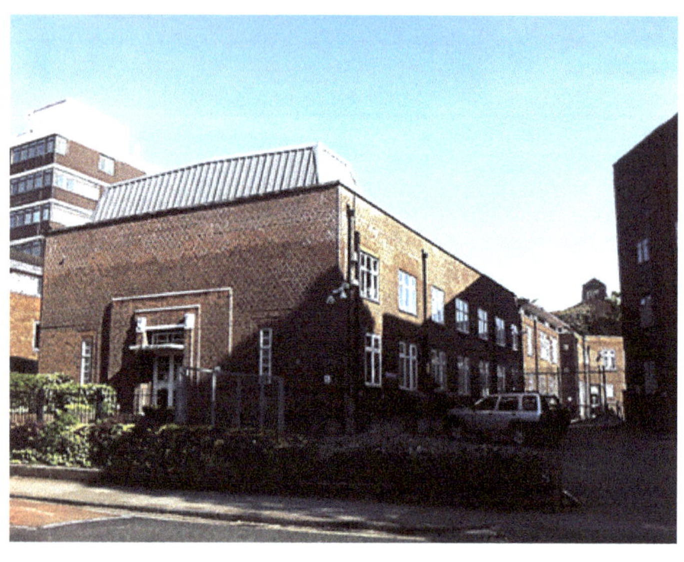

Maudsley Hospital Front Entrance

CHAPTER THREE

MAUDSLEY HOSPITAL 1959–1961

1. Settling In

My first memories of the hospital came with my parents and I visiting the hospital shortly before my admission. This visit almost definitely served a purpose with my parents speaking to the doctor in charge, a Dr C, and discussing in depth my present circumstances ahead of my admittance on 26th November 1959.

In between, I was still at Southwold until my admission date. So around 12pm, I began making my way home and had lunch before both my parents and I started getting ready for the journey to Maudsley Hospital.

On arrival, we were met by a middle-aged contact, Miss Walker who completed the necessary formalities. Then we were shown around by a nurse. I found this procedure very friendly. Easing any newcomer into the hospital complex in the tour and introducing us to hospital staff members – specifically, Nurse D, the Charge Nurse already playing a huge role with the patients under his care, and seeing my fellow patients for the first time. With the tour in full swing, I soon became familiarised with the hospital playroom and the school opposite which was sectioned off in the breaks and unlocked when attending our classes.

At the end of the tour I was left in the company of the patients and hospital staff to get settled and, in time or at least, stopping my challenging behaviour.

In between, I was under Dr R who saw the effect the anxiety was having through separating from my family; I also felt sick, and that with the right education set-up, it may have made things easier by being kept at home as one advantage.

At this stage of my life, I hardly had any friends and, before making any new friends within the hospital community, I had to sort myself out. I was sent to the Maudsley through uncontrollable behaviour and refusing to eat properly other than biscuits; still kissing heads and playing around with people's hair. Including perfect strangers with the example given below…

At nine years of age, it appeared unusual approaching a middle-aged father during a family visit, by playing around with his hair and making an upright quiff. So, without any understanding towards my inappropriate behaviour he took into account that I was young and more likely aware that I had a form of impairment.

F or 'Fin' for short was one nurse who seemed fine when playing with his hair. I also knew that he was living in a nearby villa in the hospital grounds and decided to visit him.

As he came to the door he spoke in a very loud and friendly way.

"Hello! Nice to see you! How are you keeping!?"

It was the way he was and, feeling almost certain that he was one of the most popular among his fellow staff members, I felt welcomed by his kindness; he was one of the nicest characters that one could ever meet. Dr R, I could also 'look up to' and also, good at appeasing my mind; she too, may have had a degree in psychology, the study of people's behaviour.

In comparison to this, I continued feeling uneasy, lining up later to take Malt Extract, Cod Liver Oil. It was so revolting and enough to make anyone violently sick in the process. I may have been 'spared' this 'awful' stuff and eliminating a vomiting episode by having the necessary communication skills, and getting the staff to listen that I had an upset stomach through my nerves getting the better of me.

In this difficult period, in the late 1950s and well beyond, the medical profession knew very little about autism and the digestion disturbances affecting these people.

As an individual, other patients too had issues needing addressing. These varied from hitting each other or, unwilling to eat properly (as in my case) and many more issues. In the beginning I found that the sickness experienced earlier, was comprehensible through parting from my family and, starting a new life among my fellow patients. I could no longer attend mainstream school, so making new friends with my fellow patients was more appropriate and 'palling up' with a patient named Johnny. Sometimes, he experienced nervous episodes and was no trouble to anyone. I got on very well with him and found our friendship secure over a period of at least six months.

As my nerves were easing on my first day, I found myself 'coming to' and in a better frame of mind by changing my tune, 'skylarking around' and hitting a nurse on the head.

Displeased about my skylarking, he started hitting me back and retorting, "Next time I'll pull your pants down." By describing him – he had grey hair and looking the austere type, was bound to 'hit out' at anyone misbehaving. Once I witnessed him smacking one patient straight in the eye.

I thought this behaviour unnecessary, regardless of the patient repetitiously saying 'f**k off'. None of us reported him to the Senior Charge Nurse, Nurse D.

His actions were bad enough and some staff members were as bad and, witnessed by a former patient perceiving…

A nurse spanking a male contact for hitting someone

in the eye over a broken plastic soldier belonging to a patient.

The sister in charge pinching a patient. His wrongdoing was holding a girl and protecting himself from attack either by her, or, a violent patient.

Through mentioning these 'things', a certain element of discipline existed and mostly were less severe compared to my eventual stay at boarding school. So anyone responsible at the time, had little or no knowledge that hitting us was the answer and that I would be 'making my presence felt' later.

On the lighter side, I also heard from one former Maudsley patient that Nurse D made patients laugh by tickling them.

In general, he had the top position of authority in the Children's Department. Mild-mannered and using his authority wisely as well as understanding. Including reassurance to my family that I was fine under his care and, a duty by informing my parents about any signs of relapsed hyperactivity.

Through being a little 'playful' earlier, I became quiet and unwilling to socialise. I felt that my confidence was lacking and needing extra time settling into the hospital's routine before composing myself better.

As we were winding down for the night, I lay on my pillow observing what was going on. Picking up on two names, Brian and David before getting rid of any anxieties with a well-deserved, good night's sleep.

At 7.30am, we were woken by the staff members and I felt much better; any nervousness I had, by now, was gone. I had breakfast as normal and 'time out', playing or socialising in an enclosure called 'The Garden' and still thinking to myself…

'Why my fellow pupils or staff members gave the enclosure this name appeared strange; the strange and ironic thing, that it had a sand pit, paddling pool and a couple of trees. One can understand the trees, the paddling pool and sand pit however is part of a children's playground!' So I tended to end up saying to myself, "How does all that add up!?"

Following breakfast and providing the weather stayed dry, we were often seen playing around in this area and, as before, getting into further trouble. This time by throwing scraps of wood lying around with a stray piece accidentally hitting a patient. Feeling far from pleased she started hitting me in the process. She was one of a few, accepting no nonsense and the type taking action 'when push came to shove' as the old saying goes.

Before getting into a few 'scraps' myself, I refrained from retaliating by hitting her back; by doing so, I may have been seen ending up as the 'fall guy' and/or coming off worse.

Once recovering from the incident, time was getting near to attending the hospital school for the first time; the classes were small and catering for about 15 patients in each and run separately by two teachers, Mr S and Miss M. I had Miss M throughout my stay who taught me to divide numbers; these were relatively simple and believed that my previous school (Southwold) could have included this requisite in their curriculum.

At the age that I was, my education and social skills had to improve or I would experience a lifetime drawing benefits, taking menial dead-end jobs and resulting in no real future prospects coming my way. So I must have felt compelled adapting to this set-up and trying to make gradual progress.

In between lessons, we had some privileges in the offering and soon I noticed Mr S's class visiting various places in London. So, as an opportunist, asked him if I could join. I was accepted immediately and I was lucky enough to be part of the group visiting the London Transport and National History Museum.

As I felt this was a privilege joining his class. I recall this as one of my first achievements where I felt capable of ‘speaking up for myself.’ Mr S too was good at arranging other activities for our amusement. One activity he had was making ink blobs with the concept of…

Adding a few drops of ink to paper
Folding up the paper
Unfolding the paper to see the created impression.

This was one activity keeping us amused, and also we often played darts using a target or score sheet drawing with numbers; coinciding with an obsession I had about coming last in anything and failing to participate, including the last throwing the darts already in play. As I grew older, this obsession went.

Mr S and another teacher, Mr R, knew of my obsessions.

Mr R had a mild-manner about him and was often friendly. Sometimes and I’m surmising, he may have been helping out when any one of the two teachers were absent for any reason. So helping out in the school were two other staff members:

Miss T taking charge of the admin side of things.

Mr B a middle-aged woodwork teacher whose class was situated next door to the playroom.

I often attended Mr B’s classes until falling out with a nurse where he stopped me entering his class. Whatever I was supposed to have done wrong, he saw no cause for acting the way he did when re-entering his class and trying to hide behind the woodwork bench. This ploy however failed and catching sight of me, he entered Mr B’s class, dragged me out and took me to a dormitory where I was put to bed. On the way, I continued putting up some resistance towards him, getting a slap or two on the way, and in the process I could see that he was failing to listen to my pleas to be left alone.

This was the reality at the time and thought that he could have resolved things more appropriately; or, given a warning beforehand before taking any appropriate action for correcting my behaviour.

It appeared that apart from us getting the odd 'slap' here and there, this was how some of the staff members behaved, with another example being when forced to attend weekly swimming sessions and dragged to the local swimming baths. In the process, I was shouting and crying on the way for any onlookers witnessing my outbursts and failing, in comparison to today, to intervene.

Between the episodes, and each weekend without fail, I always had visits from my family where I had plenty of opportunities to mention about the behaviour of some staff members. Being that sort of child, any misgivings that I had were soon forgotten about. So in the course of the visits, I only spoke about things taking place at that time.

Sometimes, with the visits taking place, I would jump out the waiting room window, taking 'time out' in the courtyard playing with toy planes and enjoying my favourite biscuits – Choc 'O' Lait – that my family often brought along. One day. I ate too many biscuits in one go and was sick later. None of us were given anti-sickness medication and, depending on so much today, through ongoing stomach problems.

My greed, I felt may have mimicked Bulimia where the individual is characterized by frequent episodes of grossly excessive food intake, or the compulsion of excessively eating too much and more frequently.

2. Allowed Home

Before experiencing frequent episodes of stomach-related problems, one good prospect came early in 1960. Each fortnight, the staff granted weekend leave; in between, we were allowed home for the day.

My first knowledge of this sudden change, came about

by asking a nurse if I could be granted the privilege. Immediately, she knew that I was one of the lucky ones going home to see more of my family.

Today, I am still bewildered how this sudden change came about and, by the time this privilege was granted, my family were just settling into alternative accommodation.

As the weather started to improve, my father took it upon himself to maintain the garden by uprooting old plants for example and setting them alight. I eventually started to help out and enjoyed the passion watching them and other rubbish go up in smoke.

One day it started to rain and I thought about trying to keep the rubbish dry by placing a tarpaulin on top. When the rain passed, again I was lucky seeing the rubbish going up in flames.

My passion to this prospect soon became short-lived with things changing and, when changing to an incinerator – a container where one could place the rubbish before burning. However, the ironic thing about this change was that I averted throwing 'one of my tantrums'. I had as much enjoyment seeing the smoke coming out of the incinerator's chimney. And, similarly, at my previous address I enjoyed lighting fires – running upstairs and seeing the smoke coming from the chimney and drifting into the distant sky.

As part of my condition. I wasn't acting 'out the ordinary' at home, yet getting excited by getting excited making paper planes and seeing them staying in the sky longer than usual. This appeared to be another one of my passions and a phase that I was into along with some of the other patients.

In between, I continued acting unreasonably with no exception on an outing taking place at nearby Ruskin Park. I was finding it very hard trying to undo my shoe lace. The nurse, looking on saw my frustration, came to my aid and had no choice other than cutting the lace. Before this, anyone in the vicinity could clearly perceive that I was throwing one of my tantrums through the frustrations of trying to untie that knot; it too may have been part of a learning curve, where an extremely difficult situation is judged accordingly and, giving up when meeting impossible tasks, including the knot that wouldn't undo!

Between any excitement and hyperactive episodes, I felt homesick through leaving my family and I was finding this intensifying since my weekend leave started. Nearby, a patient saw that I was looking subdued and tried appeasing my mind. One weekend however, his leave was stopped through misbehaving and relieving his frustrations; he ran up and down the corridors a few times. On recollection, he seemed a sincere friend, or should I say, 'a true friend'? His name was David.

In between the 'lows', I was hyperactive myself and doing the same as David. This time with a nurse called Val present and a very fast runner by any standards. Suddenly! I 'bolted', or, 'made a run for it' with Val in hot pursuit and almost grabbing hold of my clothing. My aim was trying to run to outrun Val to the end of the corridor when 'out of the blue' two workmen were making headway in the opposite direction to finish decorating the upstairs dormitories.

The fun had to end instantaneously or I would have run into them. With such limited distance, I had little time 'jumping' out of the way. Val, still in pursuit, had the opportunity of catching up and ending my mischievous behaviour before being taken back to my fellow patients nearby.

Today however, and thinking back, I still find this incident funny by going into 'overdrive' with Val giving chase. With the way I was, I was often acting up through autism or putting my boisterous activities down as mischievous for any kid my age.

By any standards, if there was anything I did that was incredibly funny, it was getting hold of a puppet and ripping out its artificial hair. Looking so different,

I just had to laugh. So, in between the mischief that I was getting up to, I was no angel; and for 'kicks' hitting some patients and, at times, making feeble excuses for my actions; getting involved with an incident involving two other patients was seen as unwise.

One day, I saw a patient involved in a fight with the perpetrator over an allegation that he stole something off him, and failing to think ahead, I too got involved by hitting the perpetrator responsible for his wrong doing.

Nurse D, who happened to be on duty required an explanation; very foolishly, I lied to Nurse D that he stole something from me. He abstained from necessitating what the stolen item was or I could have been put in an awkward position trying to explain myself.

Once confronting my fellow patient and I, we were let off without any further action taken, as in the example by being put to bed for the rest of the day.

Very soon things were getting back to normal and with the Easter holidays upon us I found it to be a very happy occasion. The year was 1960. So with Easter falling on the weekend of Friday 15th April, I was so looking forward to spending time with my family.

The weather that day, was sunny ahead of my family coming to pick me up to take me home. Everything, it seemed was going my way. I was now into pop music, and a huge fan of Cliff Richard too, with the teenage girls besotted with him and, coinciding with his latest song, 'Fall In Love With You'; also worth mentioning is 'Cathy's Clown' by the Everly Brothers –today still getting much airplay.

So, with these songs coinciding throughout the Easter break, I could forget about the hospital for a few days and settle back into family life. Staying on top form in this period was fantastic until Easter Monday when things were about to change ahead of returning to the hospital; things seemed unfair that with a short break lasting only 4 days, it had to end so soon.

Now homesick, I was lying in bed, with David reminding me of his method of cheering himself up – running up and down the corridors. He was always good at putting his fellow patients at ease. His reminder, this time round, appeared to work and I gradually stopped crying.

While everyone else around me was appearing fine, I should recount that it seemed so sad that I had to return to the hospital. So by not having autism and when, in 1960, it was safe for children to play outside, I still envisage (or imagine) local children associating with each other on such a fine end to Easter as in…

Taking that early evening stroll around the local park.

Playing outside in the street with friends, etc.

With the Easter break over. My troubles were beginning in a different light; things were going from bad to worse. Feeling sick first thing.

3. Sickness at Meal Times

Nurse D, the Senior Charge Nurse started noticing that I was taking longer than usual finishing my food and was none too pleased seeing this problem coming to light.

My eating problems were the beginning of what was to come; I soon experienced that nauseating sickness first thing in the morning and occasionally, 'throwing up' and, losing weight in the process through having nausea. An involuntary impulse to vomit.

Nurse D and his staff were unaware of this. None, so it appeared, knew about certain foods capable of upsetting some individuals. Then the same rings true with certain autistic individuals where digestive and/or bowel conditions is also common. Now more is understood about the digestion system where a fine tube is passed into the stomach for finding the causes.

"Why?" I am saying to myself, was it that any understanding was lacking about certain additives playing a role in hyperactivity and digestive disturbances and common also about…

Too much acid building up inside at night and inducing that sickness feeling first thing.

Today, there are better drugs able to reduce that sickness feeling, and saving the trouble with some individuals trying to disperse food down the toilet with nobody around. While I managed to accomplish this, I got 'caught out' throwing food out of the dormitory window by a nurse coming across bits of fried bread while in the treatment room downstairs. I found him disrespectful and would have respected him more by getting to the root cause of my eating problems, where I could have told him outright.

By taking me seriously enough, I could perceive him having the courtesy of speaking to Nurse D or the hospital doctor in charge of my case notes. By abstaining and unbelievably, I intentionally asked the same nurse about the consequences of weighing two stone. He replied in an ignorant and facetious way and in a contrived remark that I would be put on a feeding bottle. Unperturbed, I am perceiving this as plain ignorant or making a sick joke out of the predicament that I was already in. For a nine-year-old child, the dumbest individual should see this as derogatory or insulting.

Throughout the episodes of morning sickness, I found eating breakfast off-putting first thing. I could no longer have breakfast with my fellow patients and was sent to the sick room. There I was made to eat and force fed on the odd occasion or two. With lack of understanding by the staff, I also saw a nurse standing over me ensuring that I refrained from pulling any further 'fast ones'; including throwing food down the toilet or hiding some of the contents under a mattress.

As I was about to throw up, I knew that by succeeding I had to eat an extra portion of food; so I had to refrain by swallowing back the offending contents with the nurse interjecting: "You've been wasting food. This time, you're not getting away with it." This method of consuming extra food, when one has already been sick, is always unwise. One day another nurse, who should have known better, gave a second helping of cornflakes through me 'throwing up'.

With any common sense, my morning sickness could have been investigated and taking into account, any disliking for certain foods or the condition Anorexia Nervosa.

Nurse D was often involved and could have seen him obtaining a referral from the hospital doctor to King's College Hospital (opposite the Maudsley) for a routine investigation and, as mentioned before, by placing a camera inside my stomach. Had this occasion arisen, then Nurse D and his team would have had no choice acting accordingly by finding the causes of my morning sickness.

Apart from any hospital referral, a dietician is another option worth trying to find the root cause of my condition, and in a very concise example…

Foods containing too much sugar, rich plain milk and fatty foods.

On most occasions, I was allowed to have my midday meals in the dining room and occasionally, allowing me to 'get out' of eating under the presence of new staff members. Sometimes however, some patients 'put paid' to this, informing them that I had to finish whatever food items that I was trying to get away with.

Nurse D however was taking a dim view by catching me trying this ploy; by knowing about my vomiting episodes, he had a different view of giving extra food when I was generally, 'throwing up'. His decision was sensible to the point of probably putting his fellow staff members to shame.

As well as me, at least one other patient with eating problems was Marnie; she was thin herself and may have been anorexic…

> An eating disorder making people lose more weight than is considered healthy for their age and height. Persons with this disorder may have an intense fear of weight gain, even when they are underweight. They may diet or exercise too much, or use other methods to lose weight.

This statement and where I stood, was immaterial, applying to individuals worrying about their weight and often sick following an episode of binge eating.

Marnie was meaning well and proposing in a nice way, that I had to eat and at the same time trying to overcome her eating problems. My condition may have been seen as similar to an anorexic with an exception by disfavouring certain foods including, avoiding where possible: scrambled eggs, kidneys and Malt Extract Cod Liver Oil and foods containing spices.

At supper time, my stomach problems almost diminished with no sign of sickness in sight to worry about; sometimes, too attaining second helpings. By perceiving (seeing) this irony, the staff were a complete failure, with none trying to find out the root causes.

At best, they saw that I was faring well at supper time, compared to first thing before breakfast and dinner. "So why?" I am saying to myself, "it never occurred to them to have the stomach problems investigated at Kings College Hospital."

Soon however all this was to change about one year on with the morning sickness gradually disappearing. When I felt well enough, I returned to have breakfast each morning with my fellow patients.

With this improvement, it was supposed to be helping my process of leaving the Maudsley for good – or so I thought?

As I started thinking that my stomach problems were completely over, I had a setback. I was over the discomfort of feeling sick first thing; then, at supper time I had a severe stomach ache and Nurse D and a staff member seeing that I was in a bad way, made a quick and sensible decision by sending me back to the sick room.

Nobody knew the cause of my stomach pains and I can only surmise this as lacking in fluid or severe gastritis. The hospital doctor when summoned, found no cause for concern and took no further action; and I was left in the sick room to completely recover.

Today, much more is understood about how autism affects the digestive system. Including, the stomach and intermittently, making too much acid at night. Today many online articles on digestive and bowel complaints associated with autism exist including an online article – 'Autism and Digestive and Bowel disorders'.

With this incident passing, I did have a couple more episodes of sickness before leaving. However, I was very gullible and still getting up to much mischief with some friends throughout my stay. So, by mentioning the incidents unfolding in the next chapter, it may give an insight into further research by researchers specialising in psychology – the study of people, and, autism.

4. Taken In

Apart from feeling sick most days, I found myself getting into a few 'scraps' with some patients; in theory, I was always seeing myself as non-violent, easily led and 'picking fights'. Jack, a patient, was a fine lad and always challenging the staff when unable to get his own way; often arguing with flashes of temper and, unlucky enough, was brought up in a Barnardo's home. Positively, he did have plenty of toys to play with.

Appearing so young and immature for my age, I now feel that common sense should have played a part, avoiding any conflict.

Eluding the aforementioned thoughts, I was saying to my fellow patients, "Watch me have a fight with Jack." As the fight progressed, I soon became the 'fall guy'. So, nursing my bruises, I felt fortunate enough, avoiding any further harm to myself. By learning my lesson, I had no further fights with him.

Whether my motives were trying to impress the fellow patients, I failed in my actions. For Jack, it was no picnic with his 'temper tantrums' or 'paddies' when things didn't go his way. On good days, he was very pleasant and not the kind looking for any trouble.

In between the lulls in my behaviour, I could relate to my fellow patients with odd behaviour episodes with the following two out of the ordinary:

One night, I was lying in bed with a bad headache and giving one patient the opportunity to fart in my face. Standing in front, he had his a**e in front of my face with him telling me to listen before letting out a fart and inviting me to sniff. So being the fool I was, I put my face to his a**e and sniffed what he had just done. By any standards, this remained far from normal and any kind of fun should be done in a less disgusting way. Then aged 9, I never knew any better as in this next instance.

Sometimes, the fun we had was at the expense of others. Including certain staff members taking a dim view with us barricading ourselves in a dormitory side room. This process was relatively straight forward and only involved putting a bed behind the side room door.

Looking on were the staff feeling literally helpless and had to 'sit and wait' before eventually ending our misdemeanours or wrong doing.

In between, and for anyone desperate, a nearby sink came in handy for urinating in, or, a horizontal 'flap' window for doing our 'business'; the only thing missing however was the toilet paper and putting it less crudely. In addition, the running water also came in handy for cleaning ourselves up.

In the course of the fun that we were having, we socialised normally. Knowing full well that messing around, or 'winding up' the staff was risqué. To us, we were at the age and unaware of the consequences coming before us. I was one patient with odd or eccentric behaviour. Maudsley was for anyone with behaviour issues and neurological conditions, including autism. I felt that I fitted in well with most of my fellow patients in this episode, clearly seeing the staff looking on helpless.

As time was progressing and, to the relief of the staff, we decided on ending our fun and escaping any punishment in the process. We were lucky this time round and two weeks before leaving Maudsley, I was easily led by running away with a group of patients jumping over the garden gate. So finding this too good an opportunity to miss and a break from the 'same old' hospital routine, I decided to follow.

As usual, we were associating in the 'Garden' play area and watching some patients climbing over the play area's gate I soon decided to follow but only getting as far as the hospital gym. Then I started 'throwing up' in a nearby dustbin remaining out of view from the hospital. I could see this as a good thing, with it preventing us getting caught earlier and brought back to the hospital's grounds.

Soon after recovering, we continued on our way, ending up at Clapham Common. Feeling part of the crowd clearly meant enjoying this mini adventure and feeling a sense of freedom. And, compared to escaped prisoners breaking out of jail and breaking the monotonous cycle that they must endure as part of their sentences.

The police may have been unaware of our disappearance and for us it was seen as a privilege. No CCTV cameras existed to end our fun much sooner than expected, with the police taking us straight back to the hospital and handing us back to the hospital staff.

To us, we were having fun and I was foolish enough taking part until all but two of us decided on returning to the hospital grounds. On arrival, the hospital porter confronted us and, giving chase, he succeeded in catching and taking us back inside the hospital – with the exception of two lucky kids staying out until the early hours of the morning before 'calling it a night' and returning to the hospital.

By the morning, Nurse D, or a staff member, refused to let us get dressed; for the rest of the day, we had to stay in our pyjamas and were asked to clean the dormitory windows to pass the time. When everything got back to normal, things stayed that way until leaving Maudsley and progressing to a residential school in Buckinghamshire.

The hospital doctors, seeing my steady progress for themselves, decided a leaving timescale with the first review coming in June 1960. They suggested a time period of several months so, by making steady progress, I finally left the hospital on 30th June 1961.

5. Summing Up My Stay

My experience at the Maudsley came as an improvement and the beginning of integrating with patients and making at least a couple of friends on the way. One of them, Johnny and the other Danny, whom I am in touch with today as well as two former autistic patients, with the irony that their names were also Danny.

Also, as a result through the Maudsley and with staff guidance, my behaviour improved to the point in seeing my parents and Norma (my sister). We were more of a united family and getting on much better at home.

Since leaving the Maudsley, changes have been taking place there, the first of these coming in 1990; I visited the Children's Department and saw the changes for myself.

Before requested to leave the premises by the hospital porter, one change I noticed in the 'Garden' play area was the absence of trees; at the time, I was a tomboy, and always enjoyed climbing one of the trees in my latter stay at the hospital; the concept of this came by climbing a rope ladder to get to the first branch and progressing until eventually reaching the top.

Another change also eventually came with the Children's Department moving to The Bethlem Royal Hospital in Beckenham, Kent. Nurse D, before his passing, worked there when he was needed.

In place of the Children's Department at Maudsley, is the Michael Rutter Centre specialising in young people, from the age of 18 with psychological problems. Some of these could range from eating disorders including Anorexia Nervosa, Bulimia, food refusal and seeing young people suffering from depression.

In concluding this Chapter, I wish to have a final say on Nurse D since catching up with him in the early 1990s. In passing conversation, he 'touched on' that for some, it was never a happy time for many patients. This however was theoretically true and in the earlier period, it was hardly ever a happy time for me. Things however did improve before leaving where I ended up enjoying myself at the Maudsley; however, as the saying goes, 'All good things must come to an end.'

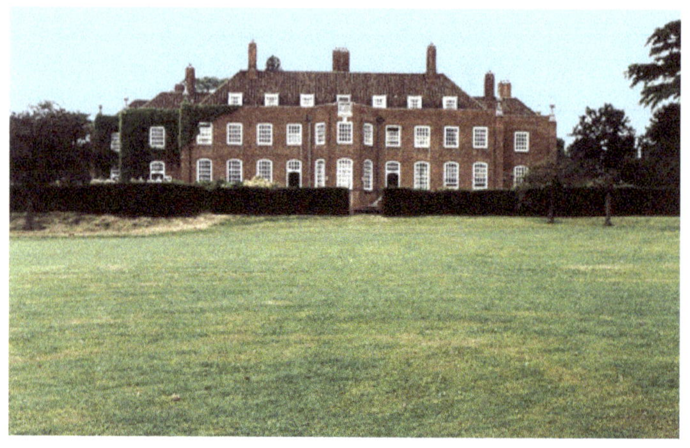

Stockgrove Park School

CHAPTER FOUR

PART ONE

BOARDING SCHOOL

A Concise Summary Of My Educational Needs

Throughout my life, Autism has ruined or blighted my life through the lack of understanding of the condition. So I am writing about my experiences, that lessons might be learnt by a cross-section of the population, including doctors and the various research bodies up and down the country.

With my time at Maudsley Hospital ending, the Educational Authorities felt that a residential school, reflecting on my circumstances, felt right. They came up with Stockgrove Park, situated in the County of Buckinghamshire, catering for…

> Pupils with special needs, including autism
>
> Families constantly moving
>
> The age criteria however was from 10 to 16 years of age.

So, at nearly three months since leaving Maudsley Hospital, I started a new life at an all-boys' boarding or residential school.

When sent by the authorities, I realised that at 10 years of age I was the youngest student, at first feeling discontented about this and failing to realise that obtaining a decent education was for my own good. But the good thing about being sent to residential school was that it saw me falling short for a 'target' for bullies in normal mainstream schools. There, some students were bound to have none or very little understanding of autism.

Eventually, once a certain amount of time had elapsed and failing to realise that I had any such impairment, I got to hear about autism for the first time in the spring of 1964 through family friends with an autistic son. He had the most unique requisite – he could easily assemble large jigsaw puzzles in full and, more than likely, in a shorter time scale than the average person.

At 13 years of age, when I first got to know their son, I considered myself an average kid until the age of 16, when I got to realise that I was a slow learner or classified as ESN (Educationally Sub Normal). Today the ESN phrase is classed as a Specific Learning Processing Difference (SLPD) and sounding much better.

Before leaving school however, and with reference to SLPD, our teacher gave us a set of complicated maths problems that we were unable to solve. And, making him realise that we were slow learners in Maths and English, he felt compelled coming up with a more simple method. He must have thought that we were on par or, as good as normal mainstream school students and unaware that some in my class, were also slow, or were slow learners like me.

In theory, I gradually found the school curriculum, or as a course of study, easier compared to most schools up and down the country. While all of this was happening, I have since made steady improvement all round. Including expressing myself better verbally, and in writing.

1. First Term

On a dull and overcast day in late September, my new life was just beginning with my family and I arriving at County Hall. Also joining were a party of pupils waiting to start a new life away from home.

On arrival, a small crowd of boys were waiting for the bus to come. I could have tried making contact with them. Yet, I felt too unhappy parting from my family and in no position making conversation either.

When the bus arrived, we said goodbye to our families before departing for the 1½ hour journey to the school. So, with the bus ready to depart, I was left with a crowd of at least 6 lads and 2 adult supervisors on the coach making its way out of London to Stockgrove Park, the residential school in Buckinghamshire. When we got there, it was already time for lunch. The dining hall was a fair size where everyone, including staff members, had our meals. So this meant getting to know whoever was serving the food, much sooner.

Soon after lunch, we met the Matron, who was responsible for getting us kitted out with school clothes, including: a suit for going to church on Sundays; a pair of slippers for indoors; and boots for outside recreation etc. To a point she was strict and very professional in her job; including enough medical knowledge for treating patients and giving out medication for various conditions and, easy enough to talk to; by upsetting her in any way, would see the unlucky one receiving the 'sharp end' of her tongue or a getting good 'telling off'.

On the first day, I continued in no mood for socialising with anyone. I needed more time for myself and trying to alleviate my anxiety. Being away from home, was no picnic. So in the intervening time period we had before supper time, I picked up a comic to read. Just anything in this short difficult period, for appeasing my mind between then and, for the rest of the day.

Helping my concerns further and for anyone with a better understanding towards anyone's feelings, fell on the Matron's husband – the Headmaster, Mr P. A middle-aged 58-year-old with much awareness observing the boys under him and, ensuring their well-being; with past experience, he had the expertise working at various schools before taking his role as Headmaster in 1950.

Throughout the rest of the day, my anxiety continued to the point of feeling sick, similarly to my first day at Maudsley. Mr P, clearly seeing that I wasn't at ease, may have thought that my anxiety precipitated a panic attack, or just feeling 'plain sick'. So, seeing the state that I was in, he tried appeasing my mind further 'over' my Marmite sandwiches and 'chasing down' the contents with milk. Seeing too that I was the new boy, that I was able to see his true kindness besides anyone else with similar problems.

With my anxiety showing, I was taking a little longer than usual by finishing off the contents. Once ready, I began making my way upstairs and shown by the Housefather (or Housemaster) my allocated dormitory, and noticed everyone laying out their clothes (or kit for short). Once this was accomplished, we had to wash and brush our teeth ahead of free time before bedtime.

By the following morning, the weather showed no improvement; still dull and overcast by the time we were awoken at 6.45am by a staff member on duty; at weekends, the wake up time was later at 7.15am.

Almost immediately, with the wake-up call in play, I found that we had to start making our own beds; with no experience accomplishing this I had to learn. In time, I learnt the skills of bed-making to an exceptional standard and enough to earn extra marks on our mark cards that we were given each week.

Before breakfast, an extra chore entailed cleaning and each of us were allocated our own Early Morning

Cleaning jobs. Mine entailed sweeping and dusting the bottom corridor.

When done very well, the full marks were…

2 for making our bed

4 for Early Morning Cleaning

2 for laying out our kit.

By the time we finished the cleaning, it was almost time for breakfast and lining up in single file. We were waiting for the gong to sound and enter the dining room for our first meal of the day; with breakfast over, it saw us lining up in the corridor before cleaning our boots and, for the remaining time, socialising in the day room; writing home, chatting away, playing games / records, listening to the radio etc.

Sometimes before making our way to our respective classes, Mr P conducted assembly and, in the process, talking about events happening at the present time or over a certain period.

Still in my memory is Mr P's nobleness for holding a special assembly for finding and handing in money. So, for many old boys who were under his care, he will always be remembered as a Father Figure for the less fortunate. Including anyone with an uncaring parent, a broken home or anyone with a disability like autism as one example.

Another staff member, Mr O, was the Deputy Teacher who recommended that I should be placed in the bottom form or, Class 4, and felt that this was the right choice under the given circumstance or, where I stood.

Through his decision, it saw an easier start, keeping up with the work and taking into account the troubles that I already had; the class I believe, had no more than 16 pupils and taking the class, was a middle-aged teacher, Mrs Ode; at other times, a male teacher took the class.

He was a disciplinarian and, in a concise form, firm yet not exactly strict.

Through anyone with similar needs to myself, I thought that 16 was a good number for anyone with a learning difficulty as any teacher can allocate more time to his or her pupils. Mrs Ode, however, preferred naming her class as, 'The Remove', probably thinking that it sounded better than 'Class 4'. In the first two terms, the Remove too, was the right class for catching up on learning various subjects, including the **three R's** –**R**eading, W**r**iting and A**r**ithmetic as a learning difference needing to be addressed before progressing further to other classes.

2. The Learning Curve

In time, I started making steady progress reaching the 'top form' of Mr O's class – Class One. Taking account of my circumstances, I may have been one of the lucky few persevering enough by reaching his class. And possessing a high enough IQ, may have helped in achieving my goal.

Usually in term time Mr P, regardless on the level of intelligence his pupils were, always arranged an IQ test, or a selection of intelligence tests. The person responsible, an invigilator, asked pupils various questions on Maths and General Knowledge. One of the lucky ones obtaining a high enough score and progressing to higher education was a lad, Gerald, achieving this; in theory and generalising a wider spectrum and 'talking out loud':

> "The idea of sending someone to main-stream school is inadvisable for anyone in my circumstances and taking into account, the following scenarios…
>
> Bullied through acting incompatibly, acting strange or, failing to 'pick up the

> cues' by saying or doing things out of place. Also, autism is a lifelong disability where, most social skills need to be learnt.
>
> Attending a mixed school, may be as bad; in some cases, besotted with jealousy through seeing any fancied female contact with a partner; and, imagining the real scenario by staring and acquiring a bad reputation in the process among fellow peers."

The other scenario could mean, trouble keeping up with the class. Gerald however, if successful and with an IQ of 92, may have found himself obtaining work more easily.

Either I may be seen as biased, or, unable to emphasise enough, the scenarios arising. So, any parent should take this into account before sending anyone with an impairment to an unfamiliar institution with lack of understanding around disabilities.

In my circumstances, I had a 'head kissing' habit; in any school outside catering for special needs, this may have been seen as odd, excluded from various activities and/or, having no friends.

With Stockgrove being a special school, besides catering for those whose families were constantly moving, an element of leeway was made as an exception. One lad, Steve, a neuro-typical easy-going lad was no exception to this rule by messing around one night before the final recreation period. He knew what was coming and, was up for some fun.

At the start of my misdemeanour, he immediately tucked his head under the bedclothes and probably was laughing at my expense; I felt lucky by facing any embarrassment with this habit; including, putting on report for the whole school to see as in…

Feldman - Kissing Steve on the head.

As I continued this habit, I recall one incident with one lad and compared to Steve, he wasn't forthcoming, with a completely incompatible view about my habit. I perceived him as non-violent unless called upon to fight and, apart from the odd fall out, we were getting on well until, one day back in 1964, I tried the same thing with him.

Suddenly, and getting the chance to steal another 'head kiss', he retaliated by jumping up and butting me in the mouth. So feeling deterred from trying the same thing for a brief period, I was soon resuming the habit of head kissing as we were lining up in single file ready to enter the dining hall.

Unaware of what was coming, I resumed kissing him on the head which, in doing so, resulted with the staff member in charge asking him having to stand behind ahead of a short lull arising from any further wrongdoing. Then I broke wind as we were lining up to enter the dining hall. So it resulted in the Housefather in charge with no choice placing him elsewhere.

With the prefects lining up separately, he may also and as a form of punishment, been put to shame by standing alongside them.

Things, so it appeared, saw that I was on a 'learning curve' and free from any shame or embarrassment on my part. Many were now aware of my eccentric behaviour and sometimes acting out of the ordinary including making silly comments about a lad with blond hair. Talking out loud on the lines such as, 'What a blond' or 'you have nice blond hair' and kissing his head too.

Each time I acted silly with him, he mainly 'played down' my own stupidity. Sometimes, when acting sensibly and compared with many teenagers, we were both into pop music. I was a fan of the Dave Clark Five. He, along with his brother and for a short period, enjoyed listening to Billy J Kramer. With both brothers anyone could have sensible conversations with them.

Most kids however can act a bit silly at times. The

'blond' lad, I felt, fitted this criteria and for this purpose on one school journey to Broadstairs, Kent…

That first day, we were associating at a swimming pool on a trip to Broadstairs and camping in the grounds at Bradstow School, Kent. Observing from a short distance, I saw this same kid, along with two other lads, chatting to some girls. Out of the blue, his words were, "He's got hairy legs." So, making light of things and being my age at 14, I could see this as a normal comment and failed taking his remark seriously. I could have said, "Yes. They can see that I've got hairy legs."

In between the period I was at Broadstairs, I felt that I was gradually maturing; at 15 years of age, the head kissing started diminishing and applying with two of my other sisters, Josephine and Barbara, about a year or so later.

One exception did remain to this rule – being unintentionally rough towards Josephine and, making society understand, that I was at the time very young and unaware of my actions.

I felt obliterated and unable to remember the temporary harm that I was doing towards her. According to her, I sat behind her and pulled her hair into agonising styles and unintentionally pulling harder or flattening her hair until achieving my required goal. Because I was completely unaware what I was doing, she had to be treated for a nervous twitch from which, thankfully, she fully recovered. If not, then it may have had a detrimental effect on me once reaching maturity.

Over a period of time, I was accepted as a 'proper brother' with the negative side of things turning into the 'positives'. Josephine started fussing and, sitting on my lap, kissing and trying to cause embarrassment in front of the rest of my family. Norma was as bad or, worse, by 'slobbering' over my face.

In addition, I was messing around with Josephine and Barbara. Chasing them round the house, and kissing their heads on catching up; plus tickling them; squirting water with a water pistol etc. It was absolute 'mental' at the time and more boisterous compared to the failure in trying to be Josephine's hairdresser? So, when something of this kind has a happy ending, it is profitable compared to families disowning their children, or as in the example with sisters, including any long-term effect that Josephine may have been having through playing with her hair too excessively.

In my teenage years I appeared unaware of what I was doing and the effects it was having on certain types of individuals.

Adding to this and my final point…

By proving things – parents should learn from this by witnessing any uncertainty about their children's eccentric behaviour.

So far, I have mentioned my weirdness with the head kissing that was more of a compulsion than autism and in comparison, as I was fussy with my sweets, I could perceive this as playing a part in my autism.

Each week my mother was always sending parcels containing comics/magazines and sweets and was very fussy when…

> Parting with extra sweets to anyone doing a good turn or making me laugh.
>
> None for anyone showing disrespect.
>
> None for the Roman Catholic minority.

All these points may seem funny, facetious, or, at the higher end of the scale, patronising. I did however have a reason for this odd behaviour and, when it came to depriving my Catholic peers of my sweets.

Each Sunday, they went to their own church in the school bus; the rest of us, whatever our Christianity, were denied this privilege. I was finding the good 3 miles or so to our own church there and back, taxing and often with tired aching feet.

I thought it unfair that the minority in the Catholic religion had this privilege, being driven to church; my fellow peers however appeared to be putting aside my concerns and that it was impossible trying to get out of going to church each Sunday.

With our vicar retiring through ill health in 1965, we endured longer walks than before. Sometimes as a rough estimate, covering 7 miles along countryside lanes. For almost a year this lasted until a new Headmaster started taking Mr P's place.

Once taking over, we no longer had to accomplish any long walks; the Roman Catholic minority still had to be taken to church.

The 'boot was now on the other foot', with the privilege of swimming, associating on the field, and 'relaxing to our heart's content'. Seeing this change felt like a sense of freedom, lounging around on the school field, listening to the latest songs on my transistor radio etc.

Also, the other good prospect came when getting better marks (as already mentioned) for…

Making our beds.

Early Morning Cleaning (EMC).

Rearranging our clothes (kit) at night.

I saw this as a start in making slow but steady progress and further progress throughout my school stay; one exception however did exist. The uncalled-for discipline criteria that many of us had to put up with.

3. Discipline

With the Christmas break complete, I had a repeat of feeling homesick. Taking the 'edge' of my homesickness,

I was soon phoning home each week; when allowed outside on my own, the choices on offer were…

> Visiting Leighton Buzzard town centre in neighbouring Bedfordshire.
>
> One of the many routes on offer; routes 1 to 5.

Taking advantage of the privilege, I found myself going further afield on my own which must have been seen as an achievement. Sometimes, and depending on the disability and severity, one could be much older than 11 years of age before having the confidence venturing out on their own.

I felt lucky and finding the routes pleasant enough and able to remain at peace with myself through the peace and quiet of the countryside and, with well-deserved exercise. Swimming also was also another pastime. The discipline however was strict and resenting certain staff members getting heavy handed; sometimes this was the only way of keeping us under control.

My autism appeared a failure by thinking along the lines of the 'normal kid on the block' (as the saying goes) and classed as naughty. The word 'autism' was misunderstood by anyone associated with Stockgrove, including the PE teacher with little or no knowledge about the condition.

Whatever wrongdoing that I was supposed to have done, I was threatened with the slipper and asked to bend over in the process.

I knew what was coming and knowing the degree of pain, I interjected with… "I know what you are going to do." Immediately, he could see that I was unhappy with what was coming and, as an alternate punishment, I was made to stand in a corner with my hands on my head.

So, going ahead with his intentions may have made me feel resentful and eventually, taking it out with my family. As always. **Hitting is NOT the answer**. The PE teacher and most staff members failed seeing this and, with no idea of any eventual psychological harm caused to some individuals.

On recollection, his way of disciplining us being that he may have been better off leaving the teaching to a teacher showing more respect or, with a rumour going around that he owned some cows in a nearby field, that attending to them may have been the better option compared to teaching in class or in the gym.

With the communication skills I had, I was unaware that these were limited and could have seen this individual acting more leniently; so too, could the staff in charge for punishing us for talking in the 'quite half hour' between 8.30 to 9pm. This time, with the prefect reporting my wrong doing, I saw no escaping the slipper this time round.

On the prefect's return, I felt compelled making my way downstairs where I found a waiting staff member, finding out soon enough what was coming and taken to a nearby classroom.

On entry, I had to take off one of my slippers before getting several strokes across my backside. When he finished, he finally demanded that I should spend the night in the classroom; hearing out his decision, I pleaded with him against taking his line of approach.

Giving in to my plea, he dropped the idea. In general, he was fair until taking a disliking to our behaviour and turning very nasty to the wrongdoer. One day I was shouting so loud when tormented by a contact, that he came down the stairs and belted the one responsible around the head; on other occasions, I screamed out loud…

> "Stop itttttttt!!" when anyone else I perceived as a tormenter.

I was fortunate that when getting these outbursts, I was spared from getting hit; these however stopped after a certain period, despite still having limited social skills.

As time went by, an improvement in my behaviour was 'on the horizon' along with any obsessions. In the early days, I was often reported by the prefect (or dormitory monitor) for talking, with the regular Housefathers dealing with the matter. A one-off incident arose and I was taken aback with my current teacher getting involved.

Before thinking twice or giving second thoughts, he made his way up the stairs, entered the dormitory and I was given a couple of slaps around the head before coolly making his way back downstairs to the staff room. On recollection, he may have been 'feeling big' inside through hitting me the way he did.

His behaviour however was also 'falling down' in class, one day as we were listening to a history broadcast. About half way through, a carillon of bells were ringing oddly.

I thought this funny and, unable to refrain from laughing, I got hit a second time and immediately I stopped laughing, feeling disconcerted instead. Looking on were my fellow classmates clearly seeing him as a killjoy, with none of them daring to speak for me through fear of getting the same treatment.

In the break period I was my normal self; my teacher however could have chosen handling the situation better by requesting staying outside the classroom until refraining more easily from laughing at those 'funny bells'.

By following things through, I could see my fellow classmates giving him more respect. At nearly 11 years of age, I felt my teacher was a violent character; with things more different today. Any teacher behaving violently towards his/her pupils risks dire consequences with the appropriate action put into place including…

A severe beating from the parent of the injured party.
Prosecuted for his/her actions.

With word getting out to our families about the physical abuse, my fellow pupils and I could see him thinking twice before hitting anyone else in a hurry.

In this arduous period, discipline was commonplace and meted out by most staff members; I continue recalling my teacher also taking action over a Times Table lesson; in between, he would say to each individual "What's 12x12?" or "10x9" and so on.

When it came to my turn to answer, I was craftily hiding the card underneath the desk and glancing down, I was calling out the answers before his suspicions were aroused. So, making his way towards where I was sitting, he saw the card and retorted, "Cheating with your card, get down there!"

By meeting his request, I had to go to the front of the class, get down on my knees with my nose touching the floor and my hands underneath my legs. In short, this is known as 'kowtowing' where I had to stay for at least an hour.

In the process, my legs were aching and stayed that way until asked to get up; then given time for the aching to subside, he allowed me to sit by my desk. In the process, a bird flew in the window with my teacher trying to coax it to fly outside. He succeeded just in time with neither of us seeming amused.

With the morning break over, I joined his woodwork class where a fleet of canoes were already on show for anyone wishing to take this pastime up as a hobby. Through the way he acted, I could perceive him dealing with things differently. Including overseeing that I had my hands on the desk throughout the Times Table session and preventing any further cheating.

Already, I was finding my teacher as a strict disciplinarian and while in the middle of my comfort stop I had no time emptying my bladder, when suddenly he took hold and escorted me back to his class. He came over as patronising and shouting out aloud…

"If anyone wants to visit the toilet, then go in the break! He went afterwards!"

Perceiving this as unacceptable, must be making anyone think how he could stoop so low?

As well as my teacher's untoward behaviour were formalities that we had to adhere to, as in writing to our families each week or, correspondence was withheld as a form of punishment. So any given opinion might be seen as unreasonable. Some students may have had serious misgivings with their family, having as little as possible to do with them.

Those who did get on with their families had to avoid any derogatory comments, including any disliking about the school as a whole. So any letter writing was usually done in the day. In comparison to when we were writing anything in the 'quite half hour period' at night. Exception was taken by any of us using a pen in case of any ink leakage while writing in bed. At the age I was, I thought this absurd and defiantly continued using my pen and disobeying the dormitory monitor, or, prefect's request to stop.

When a staff member was informed, he confiscated the pen and I started making a scene by throwing one of my tantrums; my words were, "Please, can I have my pen back!? Please!!?" At nearly 11 years of age, it seemed very unusual acting like a younger child crying through unsuccessfully trying to get his own way.

When I did calm down, it was almost time to wind down for the night. By the morning however I was confined to bed with a vertigo attack. Later, I was amused by the staff member responsible for taking my pen by joking around through his reel-to-reel tape recorder. Whatever he was saying through the dormitory speakers, had me laughing. I did eventually, get my pen back.

With this incident passing. I had what was one of my

last tantrums and was soon conforming or 'blending in' with my fellow peers.

On the discipline side of things, by us misbehaving on most occasions, we either lost marks, given a warning on any action taken, or, put on report and losing part of our pocket money; so I may have been put on report for one of many reasons including…

Feldman. Out of bounds in dormitory.

Feldman. Talking during the quiet half hour.

Apart from this, we could end up getting a 'slap' or, a succession of 'slaps', more often forcing us to comply or abide by the rules.

This practice in the 'eyes of certain staff' was meant for our own good and sometimes many of us were witnessing some 'screaming' with the pain accompanied with the beatings. I was 'no angel' misbehaving. In the summer term of 1962, I was constantly on report by various staff members; I was neither proud or ashamed by having the notoriety as the third worst misbehaved kid in the school.

In this period and beyond, I was still getting the odd slap or so, whereas today any experience of abuse is now believed and whatever excuse is given, is failing to 'wash' with the authorities. Including the very common excuse, "He fell down the stairs."

None of the authorities however knew about the discipline criteria and it was starting to get worse the following term with more staff physically abusing, with one lad fighting a staff member. At the start of the fight, a second teacher was repeatedly punching him in the ribs.

I felt far from immune to any punishment coming before me. No staff member I believe, paid little attention to the following conditions…

Autism.

An individual with a nervous disposition.

The stress endured on families constantly moving.

Other doubts were, whether any staff members knew about any well-known behavioural differences as in…

Autism	The social and communication skill condition.
ADHD	Attention Deficit Hyperactivity Disorder.
Dyspraxia	An impairment or immaturity of the organisation of movement.

And more via the Internet.

For any staff members aware of these conditions, the possibility was there for each individual member acting appropriately towards us; some staff members knew about some of us lacking in education where one may have had a Specific Learning Difference, including poor reading skills and that these issues were taken into account.

Outside the role of education issues, things continued as disgraceful or uncalled for when I was seen playing around with a bar of soap by a staff member. With no hesitation, I was ordered into the boot room next door where he started talking briefly before getting hit round the head. In the process, I felt dazed before recovering completely.

This was the beginning, with a second incident arising when serving at his tuck shop and coinciding with running down the stairs in an abrupt manner, abstaining from giving second thoughts and acting silly. He closed the tuck shop and came marching down the corridor 'like a military soldier' and belted me round the ear so hard that I fell to the floor. None of those looking on dared intervene, through fear of getting badly beaten by this 'brute of a bully'.

Even more childish or petty still, came one night with the prefect reporting me for 'breaking wind'. On this occasion, I had to make my way down the corridor to face my regular Housefather accomplishing something in the day room compared to watching television downstairs.

As he was dealing with me, he was smacking my bottom several times. Each time saying, "You're looking for trouble," before asking me to kneel down in the corridor. Finally, and grabbing a hair brush, he came out the day room, produced the hair brush and in a threatening way interjected…

"Next time you do anything like that again you will get this hairbrush. Now go back to bed."

At 11 years of age, things appeared childish, getting upset over a trivial thing and putting my name down on report for 'making silly noises' and for the sake of 'relieving myself' over something coming naturally or from severe flatulence. However, I felt lucky when I broke wind a second time while everyone was asleep, avoiding the excruciating pain endured by getting that hairbrush across my backside. Michael, a kid with the same Christian or forename, was unlucky seeing him get a broom handle over his head. So with things going a 'bit far', I could see Mr P disapproving this practice.

Mr P however had his ways of dealing with corporal punishment and can see him approving the slipper, or getting one's knuckles 'rapped' with a ruler. Caning and the hairbrush that I was threatened with, were disapproved by him.

With no further incidents taking place until the following term, I was having to watch every move I made; until one day in the spring term of 1963, I was trying to find out from Mr P about a certain film showing at the local cinema in Leighton Buzzard. Making my way to the corridor, where everyone else was lining up, I was pushed so hard by the staff member meting out the discipline as described, that once more, I fell to the floor.

Both incidents, I thought, were so petty that even a 'fool' could easily pick up on this type of behaviour. Unaware of any 'full-scale' damage that his discipline tactics may have been doing emotionally. My parents thought that the discipline criterion was there to correct us.

With any emotional distress arising through these discipline tactics, it could have meant leaving Stockgrove and placed elsewhere with staff members having a better understanding for 'special needs' children. I was unable to stay at home throughout my school duration and believed that I should have been placed in a different environment where I could have had a decent education.

With Stockgrove a fairly military type of environment, that it may have worked on some pupils; to a degree, the odd 'slap or two' may have worked. I did however respect the staff when things were good; when they were bad, I understandably took a dim view as in the example when I wasn't washing myself properly.

Observing from a short distance, my regular Housefather as before came over and worked up a lather with a sponge full of soap and thought it fun washing my face and doing it in a way with the soap finding its way through my mouth and up my nose. I found this no picnic and, according to him, having little care about my feelings. As well as this, some of us were also getting hit. For some, it appeared to be doing more harm than good; and being treated no differently regardless of any impairment, including autism.

By generalising what we had to put up with. I can perceive that belting a child is no answer, and culminating in a knock-on effect throughout the rest of that person's life a reality; so, short of trying to discredit past staff members in any way, my late father had no intentions disciplining us the way certain staff members did.

Away from school and as a result of the discipline criteria, I was taking out my frustrations on him as I was on day-leave and in the process, breaking his tool box. Before taking this action, he was saying or doing something untoward and in protest, I started breaking his tool box with a hammer. Also present was my grandfather who tried and failed in calming the situation.

Things were different with Norma intervening and trying to appease my mind; by handling things differently and with things calming down. I could have tried getting my family to listen to the following…

With the strict discipline criteria at school, appearing to 'rub off' on our families, some family members may have tried changing things, or as before, sent me to a school with more understanding for anyone with special needs.

Another alternative would have been getting the local authorities involved, and getting Mr P to change things around; with this failing, then doubts may have risen about whether Stockgrove could continue as a school and taking into account, that the discipline as before, appeared to be doing us more harm than good.

Coinciding with this incident, I had a friend, Richard, and his older brother was taking us to and from school, as we were taking day leave. Sometimes his brother would bring Richard over and take us back; it was just as well going back with Richard's brother, following the first proper fall out with my father and, one of many.

On my return, my regular Housefather got to hear about the incident and I could have mentioned my resentments with each chastisement meted out by him, resulting in me 'taking things out' on my family and breaking the tool box in the process. By going that far, he may have thought this as insinuating, smacking my face and, inevitably, fuelling my resentment further.

By nature, I wasn't the violent type. Occasionally, I got into 'scraps' as most of us do in our younger days. In between, some happy times did exist and taking the opportunity, I should break things down. Proving that in between the 'doom and gloom' happier times were taking place.

4. The Lighter Side

Before 'lights out', I was making my way back from a toilet stop and found that something wasn't right, discovering that my regular Housefather had done a disappearing act and I was asking whether anyone had seen him.

With my anxiety showing, I may have wandered off to the other two dormitories on his house (or wing) asking, "Has anyone seen Sir?" Or to the extreme, getting Mr P involved. With a scenario arising, I could see much embarrassment in the process between my Housefather and I.

By abstaining from any of the options, I entered the dormitory entrance and found him lying on my bed. Suddenly, my peers burst out laughing my expense; everyone in the dormitory must have slept well that night. I had to go along with the joke and simultaneously, taken aback, or, taken by surprise.

Regardless of my autism, I took this kind of banter well. Anyone else in my position, may have entered the dormitory and laughed along with the joke. Prior to 'joking about', I found that one day, as we were changing the bed sheets one lad, Peter, who slept in the next bed asked…

"What goes on the bottom?" referring to the sheet.

"Your trousers," replied the staff member in charge.

When things failed 'cottoning on' until later in the day, I found myself having the 'giggles' over tea along with another Housefather, Mr G, laughing as well over 'what went on the bottom?'

While looking on as being normal, I could have begun falling in love with anyone I fancied at an earlier age. Hayley Mill's the actress at the time was appearing in Walt Disney's *In Search of the Castaways.* In retrospect…

She looked absolutely stunning on the cover of *Princess* and meeting her in person, I could have been very happy and with everlasting memories to show for.

At 12 years of age, I felt too young for any physical

contact with females; meaning, kissing and cuddling as one good example. Hayley was the first female that I had feelings for but in a different way – I was a big fan of hers; and I was still liking Cliff Richard. He was admired by many; so, a true fan must have ended up feeling his presence when his records were played.

So far, I have tried 'summing up' my true feelings and, through seeing the film starring Hayley Mills, attracted an 'atmosphere' in 'my own world'. Picturing in mind, her role in *In Search of the Castaways* and that stunning picture of her in *Princess* and singing 'Let's Get Together', a minor hit 2 years previously.

The other good thing about my autism and being unaware of any wrong doing for much of the time, is that I have a higher than average intelligence in certain areas; resulting in a good excuse sharing my feelings of sadness. And taking a liking for two teachers arriving in January and March respectively. The year is 1963.

As usual, with winter term beginning and settling back into the familiar routine of things, my present teacher was in the process of leaving Stockgrove for good; in the remaining period, he made use of finishing off constructing several canoes for anyone interested enough taking up the hobby.

In his place, a new teacher, a Mr C, was taking to the role of teaching. Everyone was adoring him. He knew the meaning of respect and respecting us all. My fellow classmates and I were wishing him staying permanently until less than 2 months, sadly saw him leaving Stockgrove for good.

My classmates and I knew that things were no longer going to be the same following his departure. Later, a fellow pupil, Robert, was crying his eyes out. At a very sad time for many, it didn't occur to any of us to ask Mr C to stay.

By us speaking up for ourselves, I could see Mr C extending his stay, or, consulting Mr P about our concerns, showing clearly how upset we were on his departure. Robert, I felt, was a brilliant candidate by speaking to Mr P, at the precise moment when feeling subdued in the process.

Apart from missing my grandfather, passing away when I was six years old, these were my first true feelings about missing somebody so much (with no disrespect to my late grandfather). I felt this experience was similar to a bereavement, and it took at least 2 days or more getting over Mr C's departure. I believe too, that Robert may have felt the same way as well.

As a consolation, a teacher – an Australian teacher, Mrs D, was also well respected and attractive too and was 'standing in' until the Easter break before flying back to Australia.

As we gradually were getting used to Mr C's departure, we soon 'blended in' with Mrs D's presence and found it a great asset having her has well as Mr C and taking things 'one step further'.

I felt, along with my fellow peers, that having both these contacts teaching alongside in separate classes was a bigger asset and seeing an imminent improvement in my education sooner, rather than later. And, with any big improvement to this effect, may have helped by expressing myself more coherently or clearer.

Elaborating further, communication skills I was once told, comes when an improvement is seen with education. So with two brilliant teachers, I should give my final thoughts in ending this section of the Chapter.

On a brief visit later on by Mr C, my classroom peers were pleased to see him again. And speaking further on behalf of everyone – none of us in this period, would ever say 'No' if he contemplated returning to teaching in this period alone. Both Mr C and Mrs D were the nicest that one could ever meet; everyone in my class then must have thought it a great pleasure meeting them and they were my favourite staff members at the time.

5. The New Teacher

In the summer term of 1963, the teacher taking over Mrs D's position was less forthcoming, lacking the charisma that Mr C and Mrs D already had. I first knew this individual at least 6½ months previously on a routine visit and surmising now, as putting himself forward for the teaching post vacancy in April 1963.

Before taking Mrs D's position, I happened to be in the day room one night with a staff member recording an extract from a book. Observing was this individual. In the process, he may have taken an interest in the extract, and I was getting known by him in a short space of time.

At the start of the summer term, I found myself getting to know him better but witnessed some taking an instant dislike towards him for the following reason…

One day following a trip out, after he had boarded the coach ready for the return journey, I witnessed one peer making an unfavourable remark. I was however, not in the least surprised, as I could see him coming across as off-putting, very unfriendly and leaving a sombre atmosphere as the coach made its way back to school.

Some of us however had to put up with him as our teacher; the atmosphere in our class seemed so dull compared to when Mr C and Mrs D were in charge.

On the brighter side of things, I started 'playing up' the new teacher. One day, I tried balancing some books on my head and provoking a reaction from him. He retorted:

"Get those books off your head before I bounce them off."

I answered by saying: "You can't sir, you haven't got any balls."

He retorted once more, "Stop being cheeky!!"

The class, on the whole, were unimpressed and finding my joke far from funny; I could easily have ended up getting much worse than the odd slap.

So far, when I got hit, it came when smacking my bottom

for something else I did in front of his class. In the process, I felt no pain whatever and felt an opportunity arising by 'taking the p**s out of him' further; acting childish and counting aloud the number of slaps I was given.

Through 'acting the clown', the class this time appeared to be amused. Realising that he wasn't hurting me enough, he kept the slipper in mind for next time and, soon enough, he was having cause to use it.

As usual and up to no good, I soon found the slipper hurting more. This time, finding it no easy gain, counting aloud the number of strokes delivered with the slipper; immediately on stopping, a fellow class mate George interjected quietly that I'd had 6 strokes.

By accepting my punishment, I had to conform with his ways and, getting to know him better, I soon found out that playing him up was now inadvisable.

In the autumn term of 1963, my work was falling well short of the required standard through 'skylarking' the previous term and falling behind the rest of the class. My handwriting was substandard to the point where I was compelled to rewrite a whole exercise.

Unaware that schooling was important, it appeared that I was showing little care or attention until showing signs of improvement over 6 months later. In between this period, this teacher's unpopularity too, showed no signs of improvement and was apparent when accidentally passing wind when lining up ready for assembly.

Immediately my teacher who was taking over House 3 asked, "Who was that?"

"Feldman," replied the dormitory monitor in charge.

"Feldman," the teacher replied. "I'll see you in class."

As we were entering the class, he called me over before finding myself getting hit around the head. Then, demanding that I kowtow – and as before, meaning kneeling down, nose touching the floor and hands beneath the bottom.

Five minutes later, I was told to get up and was getting

hit again. I thought this was now beyond a joke before being asked to kowtow again; by feeling inclined, I could try fighting with him through acting silly and seeing myself as the fall guy. An easy victim.

Some peers did however, 'take him on'. Tony, a reasonable enough guy until anyone tried 'crossing' him, or upsetting to the point of him taking action.

One day, Tony had a fight outside our local church. Immediately everyone was shouting and cheering. My teacher won the fight and was thinking of finishing him off further, by picking up and waving a stick. This occasion was one of many, with his unpopularity clearly showing with many contacts.

One day after visiting our local church, I recall, after my weekend leave, of him being 'set upon' by some school students; with the beating he had, it may have taught him a lesson from 'messing' with certain individuals; so leaving my teacher to recover, the party present made their way back to school.

Before the end of term Mr P sacked him from his duties. Between this period I had a mellowed out towards my teacher by lending him a weekly science magazine included in my mother's parcels.

So, on the positive side and recounting (saying) to myself…

"I must have felt that I was one of the very few, forgiving him for any past misgivings then and continuing to do so now."

6. Childhood Obsessions

In the holidays I found myself taking things in my stride and handling things differently.

With a week's holiday to Felixstowe, West Suffolk, in play, I had a one-off obsession by standing in front of a mirror trying to get a straight parting in my hair. This went on for a good 30 minutes before satisfying myself getting my parting to perfection, in between the frustration that I was having. I would not join the other guests for the evening meal until 'that parting' was 'dead straight'.

The landlady in charge had to save my meal. Both my parents should have tried 'talking me round' as this obsession was far from normal.

I had many obsessions, including listening to Housewives' Choice, Children's Favourites and Easy Beat; by missing the start of these programs, it would mean turning off the radio and waking as early as 5am the following day.

By accomplishing this plan, I always went back to sleep; so a better plan was to set the alarm at around 8.45am for the 9am start for Housewives' Choice to begin.

Towards the end of my childhood, I felt eluded by these methods; with my father trying silly games such as breaking wind loudly, and his childish behaviour failed to lift my spirits for long.

I remember this incident well…

One snowy cold January day in 1963 I overslept and missed part of Housewives' Choice and, as usual, I turned off the radio. As a joke, my mother's words were, "Shall I fart?"

Suddenly, my father 'let rip'. So, along with my mother, I found myself temporarily laughing before reverting back to my usual self. This childish behaviour seemed so silly and laughable by any standard and unknowingly without a second thought.

By making a joke of his behaviour, I was repeatedly asking my mother…

"What did Dad do in bed on January 7th 1963?" The exact date when this arose.

In this period as well we had a harsh winter, with more than enough snow to put myself to the challenge of building an igloo in our back garden and, continuing being childish or unreasonable in the process.

I was feeling determined in building that igloo. No matter what! And, unaware that it wasn't cold enough for performing my goal. Each time I added more snow, the igloo continued collapsing.

In the end, I succumbed altogether through getting in a state. Already my family were hinting that I may have better luck the following morning. By heeding their advice, I went back into the garden the next morning and succeeded in rebuilding that igloo completely.

In this same period, I tried hanging Christmas decorations in the living room using Sellotape. Sure enough, the same as the igloo, they continued falling down resulting in more frustration. There was one trick to this rule however, keeping the decorations intact – hammering drawing pins into the walls; this may have 'done the trick' and with an open fire heater in the same room, less risk of the room catching alight.

As I got older, further into my teenage years, these childish obsessions gradually started to diminish.

7. Teenage Years

On 13th November 1963, I had reached my teens. The Beatles were gaining popularity with their fans and making front page news. They were adored by their fans and unable to go anywhere when coming into contact with them.

Coinciding with 'Beatlemania', a new term was beginning and usually I was feeling uncomfortable returning at the end of the holidays, but my troubles soon disappeared that night witnessing a Beatles' period once settling in for the new term.

The year 1964 saw the new term beginning in fine style and the Beatles latest album, 'With the Beatles', was in full play.

With my autism to go by and seeing my fellow peers

very excited, it seemed ironic by any standard and witnessing this instance alone…

Some were shaking their heads, full of excitement, and fantasising by pretending to be the Beatles themselves; so short of trying to be patronising, it may have been seen as more comprehensible had my peers had ASD themselves. With common sense, I comfortably refrained from reaching their level or their moment of fantasy.

Mr P, and no disrespect to him, heard about their excitement and must have thought it a 'bit weird' with those involved getting 'over excited'. And excited my fellow peers were, with Mr P's words recounting that they were…

'Shaking their silly heads off.'

Now and using my common sense, I may have been putting my fellow peers to shame and witnessing them fantasising or 'living in Cloud Cuckoo Land' or failing to face reality.

With Beatlemania in full swing, many Stockgrove lads and I were Beatles crazy. I soon started perceiving this as something new to pop culture, with four young Liverpool lads about to change the world, meaning 'Beatle crazy' falling short of getting too excited over them.

With this radical change, the Beatles were making many people happy with their music; and crucially music for some can be a great way of alleviating any despondency, or, Seasonal Affective Disorder (SAD) in the winter months.

At school, I was free from any SAD symptoms and in February 1964, I had something to smile about with Mr P allowing us weekend leave.

Out of the blue, Mr P started announcing this scheme for the first time and resulting in a 'blessing' for the boys under his care. Seeing their families each fortnight in comparison to four weeks at a time under the old system.

Since his demise or passing, I am taking the opportunity by mentioning his thoughtfulness as the most prestigious things that he did for the boys under him and respecting him for this. In between the remaining period he had left before retiring, he may have failed to realise how many lives he 'changed around' by introducing the weekend leave scheme; helping things along too. I had caring parents, and seeing them more often was good for my morale. Right from the start, both parents were there through 'thick and thin' and mattered a lot.

Now into the early part of my teenage years, and coinciding with the caring parents I had, I was on the brink of adolescence.

8. Early Adolescence

As part of my adolescence, I was into female contacts. In between, the instances that I had was, like all teenagers – part of growing up.

One day, my family and I were at a Butlins Holiday Camp in Bognor Regis when I started taking a rowing boat out on a boating lake; I was about to get to shore when I found myself unable to handle the boat. My frustrations were clearly showing, until the people in charge stepped in by giving guidance and getting the boat safely back to shore.

Perhaps I was acting foolhardy, and I must have been unaware that rowing required a skill, or, I may have been perceived with Dyspraxia – the inability to perform coordinated movements.

With my ordeal over, I was thinking twice about going it alone in a rowing boat and only accomplishing the task with somebody.

Putting aside the lack of knowledge and keeping calm, I continued having my obsessions and often watched 'Thank Your Lucky Stars.' A 'pop' program with various acts appearing each week.

At the age of 13, I was a huge fan of the Dave Clark

Five and today, I continue enjoying their songs. And, they were to appear on 'Thank Your lucky Stars' at the end of our holiday.

The boarding house where we were staying had a television, and at the end of the program, the compère announced that the band was appearing on the next show. This was a turning point for another one of my obsessions to materialise.

When it was time to leave, I had to get home in time to see the band perform again. I was spoilt and failing to take into account how my family were thinking, contemplating extending their stay for an extra couple of hours or so; making the most of some fine overdue weather, following a dull and overcast week. It appeared typical that after a bad week with overcast weather, that it had to be fine on our last day.

With the weather warm too, my family and three cousins holidaying with us were reluctant to leave and had the desire to make the most of the glorious fine weather. I felt the opposite, and unable to think ahead of the band's future TV appearances. I continued insisting to my parents to leave early.

In 1964 YouTube was unheard of, along with video recorders and iPlayer. So the only alternative to 'catching' them performing, was on TV. My parents could easily have appeased my mind by adding…

"Look Michael, they will be appearing on television again soon."

I may have accepted their reassurance, and better for them than giving into my demands and granting my request.

On the way home, we were delayed by the constant changing of traffic lights turning red and that "safety on the roads takes priority compared to going past the 'offending red traffic lights', **No matter what**!"

With the 'offending' lights holding us up, the attempt at getting home on time failed. Turning on the TV, the band were already performing their latest song, 'Thinking Of You Baby'.

Through my disappointment and through missing the beginning of their performance, I turned off the TV. In my younger years I had these obsessions, and neither of my parents knew about trying to 'talk me round' over things coinciding and causing conflict in the process.

Giving credit, I felt that my family tried very hard getting back home in time or I may have been given the train fare home; by accomplishing this, I could see my family continuing their holiday in peace and staying in Bognor until late in the day or early evening.

Today however, many of the band's recordings are on YouTube (shown in the link) and how the band looked at the time when they were my favourite act:

http://www.youtube.com/watch?v=s3G-gCfIjK8

This link will also have the song, 'Thinking Of You Baby'.

Through my unreasonable behaviour at this awkward time, I am feeling ashamed about behaving in such a way. Besides failing to conform to my family the way I would have liked, they knew that I was a slow learner and that this separate disability was affecting me so much, that I could have foreseen life getting extremely hard at any nearby mainstream school in Hackney.

While I was disappointed that I was unable to see Dave Clark and his band from the start, I was ready to have piano lessons when becoming more settled after my disappointment. So my family arranged this through Norma's teacher, Tommy. This however was no big problem and my father introduced me to Tommy for the concept of learning to read music.

As the lessons progressed, those 'little dots' on the music sheet began making sense. I deciphered that those dots comprised of the first seven letters of the alphabet and making identical sounds. So in concise form A to G.

At least Tommy gave me that chance in time for one new activity where piano lessons were taking place in the school's new term. Throughout the new Autumn Term, learning with my fellow peers was fun, including having a few laughs along the way. One lad, John, was enjoying a good laugh playing a trumpet and finding the sounds appearing unnatural.

Since joining the music teacher's class, my interest in playing the piano increased until the lessons came to an end; my sister, Norma took over the role by giving free lessons and saved my parents a fortune in private lessons.

When getting more advanced, playing the pieces in front of me, so did my obsession. I was often playing a whole piece of music over and over and trying to avoid making one mistake; everything had to be played to perfection as if entering any music exam where the piece had to be perfect for any chance of passing the exam.

So far, by getting worked up was no way forward and, unintentionally, being rude to a staff member was also 'out of character'. Most commonly, I was often disturbed by my fellow peers, until one day a staff member was entering the classroom and 'bearing the brunt' of my outburst, I told her to "Get out!"

Taken aback on her part, I tried calming down and agreed by letting her hear the piece that I so desperately tried getting to perfection.

With the predicament that I was in, I felt 'out of reality', unable to compose myself to anyone. I felt that as well as my autism came a certain amount of frustration, including cursing or blaspheming during frustrating episodes.

Through thinking back on this episode with the piano, a better strategy or plan is…

Going back a bar or two, or part of the piece and try hitting the notes 'head on'. Taking a break from my frustrations, or trying an easier piece of music to be getting on with and saving much stress.

In time, I did outgrow this obsession and took the sensible option of taking things in my stride when things were failing to go to plan when trying to hit the right notes. So, in between hitting 'bum notes' and making a joke out of my obsessions, things were good.

Mr P too had his ways. I was entering the dining room for breakfast one day and he saw that I was 'improperly dressed' and put on report; either my shirt was sticking out too far and improperly tucked in, or, my belt wasn't properly buckled.

When it came to assembly, and still unaware of any dress sense that I had my belt sticking out, suddenly and unexpectedly in front of everybody he came out with…

"What's this? Gesticulated penis?"

When he said this, one student, John in assembly, mentioned in passing to our class, that he could not control himself laughing; also, when I tried contacting him on Friend's reunited many years back,, he too could not believe that it was me.

Already by now, I was feeling corrupted, and as usual I had my belt sticking out. Mr P's words this time were, "Tuck your dickie in" until the third time trying the same thing, the joke started getting stale and I had to stop. So as young as I was, I tried 'panning out' the joke that he was having on me.

While I may have acted a little immature at the age I was, one of my first achievements was a Bronze Medallion in Life Saving and also passing a Road Safety Cycling Course. I continued having my obsessions. As part of my autism, I tried getting filmed swimming so that I could see myself splashing about 'on playback' as one of the many film shows in the darker months.

Usually, the filming (via a movie camera) was randomly taking place throughout May to July, until learning that the Housefather doing the filming had it postponed until the Autumn; by the time the new term came, I lost this obsession together and went swimming less often.

In this time period, I felt that at 14 years of age, my life was getting more turbulent; I should have been as good as any normal kid in comparison to being in a 'world of my own'. And, besotted with jealousy with the 'chosen few' with better bodies and getting sunburnt more easily. So theoretically, some adolescents worry about weight gain or perhaps more by suffering from acne – a disease where one is covered with spots, or blotchy skin in the process.

The events unfolding in the summer term of 1965 came by experiencing my first real issue, one fine June evening with the weather warm enough for sunbathing. I was taking things far too seriously by asking one of the lads to look at my back and finding out whether it was red.

When told that I had a reddish brown colour against seeing my fellow associates with sunburn, I felt jealous to the point in getting very upset. At the time, I was perceiving this idiosyncrasy as normal.

With nobody else thinking the way I did, I have to say that seeing the lucky few alone, with superb bodies, is something to be jealous of and before taking into account, anyone with sunburn. I felt eluded that getting sunburnt was unhealthy and that a tan is much better.

So, my emotions were now running very high. Feeling depressed in the process through the fixation of getting sunburnt with no success. By obtaining a cream, enabling my skin to turn whiter, at least I could see 'half the battle won'.

By the time the summer holidays arrived, things at home were fine despite 'bottling up' my feelings. Then one day, my father upset me and I ended up by threatening him with a bottle that I already had in my hand. In surmising, I may have upset my sister, Josephine. For whatever reasons I was doing to upset Josephine, I felt it reprehensible for his threatening behaviour.

Normally, I may have tried talking my way out of the argument, or trying to get him to listen; taking into account that threatening to hit someone is no answer and that addressing the situation in a more subtle way is the better course of action.

With any subtleness, it may have helped things along by offering him an apology and better in comparison to carrying out threats and seeing the prospects of being locked up in a psychiatric hospital; many hospitals of this type existed for mental illness besides autism. They were lacking understanding to a certain degree, with many continuing 'caught up in the system'.

Today, most mental illness issues are managed in the community, including teenagers experiencing emotional turmoil in their adolescent years and ranging from…

Obesity

Too many spots (as already mentioned)

Boyfriend/girlfriend problems

And so on…

At only 14 years of age, I felt insecure and feeling 'trapped' inside, through the inevitable change of hormones appearing to play havoc and higher than the average teenager. Things too were failing to help with a selection of sentimental songs played on the radio. Including…

Leave a Little Love	Lulu
Where Are You Now My Love	Jackie Trent
Make It Easy On Yourself'	The Walker Brothers
Baby Don't Go'	Sonny and Cher
Some Of Your Loving	Dusty Springfield

With much time elapsed, these songs were coinciding badly with the exception of 'Where Are You Now My Love', a song meaning more than any other, coinciding with Betty and I getting together.

In between the timescale of late spring and summer, it may have been a good move seeing a psychiatrist with he or she getting to the bottom of things and prescribing tranquilizers for rectifying the problems that I was having.

With special schools existing in Hackney, I could confide in my parents better and in comparison with unsympathetic staff that I was having to put up with. So between this difficult period, I felt too young getting to grips with my jealousy at a peak with these individuals with very good bodies. There was another boy called Michael attending school at the same time. He too, had a fantastic body (another lucky one) who also ended up in prison later in life.

By threatening my father the way I did, my immediate family knew about respect with none of them being the bullying or authoritarian type. I often respected this and needed time trying to calm myself. Including, trying to take my mind off the first proper fallout with my father, and trying to forget the incident by playing with a gyro top in the front porch outside.

Today I am feeling ashamed of my actions and could have ended in 'deep trouble' by any harm coming to him, and sad that I was unable to handle the situation in a more subtle way.

With certain staff members counted on as untrustworthy, talking through my problems was a waste of time. Now that all have passed away, I should take the opportunity by putting certain members responsible to shame and with their actions 'rubbing off' on my family with…

Some having no sympathy and, clearly seeing how upset through failing to begin with, receiving any correspondence from my Bradstow contacts that I am yet to mention.

The physical abuse meted out by doing something to their disliking. A recipe for disaster when culminating any individual's violent tendencies later in life.

To a degree, I felt lucky escaping too much physical and emotional harm through the abuse experienced.

Now into the early part of my teenage years and coinciding with the caring parents I had, I was on the brink of adolescence and helping things further by getting to know Betty, a girl living next door to us. So with this unexpected change coming, I knew that as well as seeing my family more often, that I could see Betty at least fortnightly.

In between and with so many female contacts in my life, I shall only be mentioning anyone of significance importance and the emotional turmoil that I was to face in these time periods.

Primarily and starting with Betty. When getting to know Betty, things started off well. The beginning of what was, the verge of a relationship coming when…

One spring morning, some friends and I were setting off to see an air display at Panshanger Airfield in Hertfordshire; before setting off, I noticed Betty sitting in the front seat of my father's van and, unconsciously, I started playing with her hair. To begin with, she may have thought it relaxing; but when I started playing with her hair too often, it appeared she was feeling too uncomfortable and in the process, saying in her own words. "Go way."

This 'kink' I had with her, went on for over a year.

I thought no more of Betty until one fine May morning in 1964 when I dreamt about her, before waking up at with a 'somewhat' mellow feeling inside of me. My fellow peers (or students) were still sound asleep as I lay in my bed, constantly thinking of her for a good 15 minutes.

Before the 6.45am wake-up call, I was dreaming of Betty and guessing that she must have been happily playing in the street with friends. She seemed very happy, and sweet and innocent; since dreaming about her, I cannot recall having any further dreams of this kind.

So far, my experience appears to be common with this

'fairytale' imagination taking place; at 13 years of age, I saw this as the beginning of romance with Betty and it appeared that my autism was no barrier for stopping the romance already on the horizon.

Before romance blossomed, the elongated crush I had lasted at least a year before Betty and I were getting properly together but my autism started getting in the way of the relationship that we were having. Including, acting silly with Betty and chasing her down the street until chasing her too often and she would be bursting into tears.

Obliterated by my 'skylarking, or, refusing to stop and looking at consequences, I found myself getting less far with Betty; by saying 'sorry' may have helped getting things 'back on track.'

Her parents however were far from pleased and looking back any looming relationship may not have been so forthcoming. So, with sound advice from my own family, came no further 'skylarking' and in its place came a turning point through calming down and acting more sensibly.

With things back to normal, things started turning round in my favour.

One fine evening, my friends came round with a Scalextric set; also present were Betty and her brother, Stanley.

As soon as things were set up, we were watching the cars go round the circuit. Suddenly, I found the excitement over Betty, building up inside; by liking her more, I started having my first true feelings of love with her sitting on my lap and hugging her at the same time. With this experience arising and being the first of its kind, I continued behaving this way when in contact with any 'fancied' female – it is so 'nice', so it is appropriate reciprocating back.

With my mother looking on, she could clearly see that apart from blushing, I was also very happy and coinciding with any shyness that I may have had in the process. At only

14 years of age, this was my first taste of 'true happiness'. I also believed that with this happiness continuing for a prolonged period, that it may have completely changed my life i.e. no worrying about anyone else and saving further heartache with contacts around my age.

Through being 'frisky' or 'high spirited' with Betty in the beginning, or, in the first year since knowing her, in her own words she said that 'I wasn't the worst kid in the street'; Stanley, her brother, may have seen things in another light when hitting him through doing something to my disliking. He was the kind that showed his 'true character', and was the flamboyant type with some disapproving the way he was and getting into a few 'scraps' with kids around his age.

I can also perceive Stanley deliberately finding the slightest thing out of the ordinary as very funny. One day, Betty was holding her guinea pig with its bottom or 'rear' facing her. Suddenly, it urinated down her jumper. By Stanley witnessing this, he would inevitably laugh himself 'silly'. Poor Betty however, wasn't so amused. My fellow peers did though, when I was reciting this incident from my diary on a trip to Broadstairs when everyone fell about laughing.

With reference to this incident, Betty started teasing by holding her guinea pig with its head facing towards her. With its 'rear end' right in front of my face, she was expecting it to urinate over me; with any incident arising. I could perceive Betty, myself and her family laughing hysterically. The guinea pig however was good and knew of Betty's teasing right from the start; and, through experience, I can get upset through teasing.

I was advising Betty to refrain further from holding the guinea pig's a**e in front of my face following a fresh change of clothing. Getting hostile towards Betty was risking the end of the friendship so far with her parents, stopping further contact between the two of us.

So, refraining from going near her could mean a 'recipe

for disaster' to the point of regretting my actions and, in the process, to profound unhappiness.

So far, the Easter holiday in 1965 I thought was the happiest that I have been for a long time; as it was ending and, with showing some affection, I gave Betty a ring won at a fairground.

Through knowing Betty better, I was already calming down and refraining from chasing her along the street. In this initial time frame, she felt very special in my heart with the pinnacle of good things come.

With our relationship in full swing and with intense feelings, I was so looking forward to seeing her; in the usual procedure and before the pinnacle of our friendship, she wrote ahead of taking weekend leave. In one letter, she sent a nice picture of herself and I happened to see Mr P who was standing in for a staff member, reading one of her letters.

As I was taking 'leave', I started making my way home by catching the bus to Leighton Buzzard, walking to the station and catching the train to Euston and finally, a bus home.

In my favour, the weather was on my side and ideal for being outdoors. Betty was already associating with her friends when I came across her coming into view near the bottom of the slope. With limited social skills, I found it hard knowing exactly what to say.

Both of us were 'caught off guard', not knowing what to say to each other. I was near home and needed more time settling in before meeting with Betty that evening and, having a better chance composing myself.

Later that evening, I was succeeding in getting my act together and venturing into the street, when I saw Betty playing with an older friend, Michelle. With time going on, I spoke to Betty before lying down on a patch of grass where we started cuddling each other.

Describing my feelings, I felt ecstatic cuddling and with much feeling around as well as feeling shy, I was wishing that I could bring myself to kiss Betty. I left this up to her which she did. So, being much taller than she was, she climbed a set of railings and gave a succession of kisses with one catching my lips.

It was seemingly obvious that Betty had more confidence and less shyness compared to myself, and I would have liked to have 'brought myself' to kiss her more passionately. In passing conversation, she remembers the friendship that we had together; apart from playing with her hair or patting her on the head, I was beginning to stop when 'being together'.

With this unforgettable encounter, we both told our families about our 'love romances'. So far, I felt very fortunate having Betty, where many neuro-diverse individuals are lacking the social skills when it comes to successful integration with female company.

On the higher end of the spectrum, the 'stakes' are higher and, with the right initiative, he or she can 'hit it off' more easily; provided that he or she isn't fussy or choosy on looks. In the beginning, I wasn't choosy and very soon I was finding that 'true love never runs smooth'.

With our relationship still peaking, Betty's mood changed following a potato (or spud) throwing incident between myself and the kids that I was associating with. I felt that messing around with the older lads was nothing 'out of the ordinary', until one of the spuds caught her on the back of the leg.

Suddenly, her mood soon changed saying… "Don't like you any more."

So, the age I was, I failed using my initiative, believing that she may have been joking, and I failed offering an apology. With Betty's decision by ending our relationship so abruptly, I still felt that I had a chance with her, or now, 'living in a fantasy world' by looking at her photograph that she sent as I was lying in bed back at school.

Still living in 'fantasy land', I was unable to avoid

looking at her photograph, kissing it at the same time and stopping as it was getting too dark. Over a certain amount of time, I soon started realising that our relationship was foundering.

Through acting silly and led on by the kids throwing potatoes, she stopped sending any further correspondence; her decision or snub over the 'silly potato throwing' incident was through her age and not knowing how to handle things. Ironically, I felt unperturbed with the trip to Broadstairs very near, that any upset caused, I felt, would soon be forgotten.

Betty however and through her age, was unforgiving and, constantly finding her attractive, I was hoping to revive the relationship we had. I tried kissing her in front of her friends, perhaps embarrassing her in the process and luckily avoiding getting hurt through any of her friends taking action.

In the surroundings, or the area where I lived, I had no feelings for anyone else. So, learning by the hang-ups, I feel more the wiser by…

Giving Betty a 'wild berth' when seen associating with friends and avoiding any risk of her informing her parents about the way I was behaving.

Walking away and joining my friends, or, finding something else to do.

With time elapsing getting her parents 'talking her round' and rekindling the friendship that we had, seemed another appropriate option.

Apart from approaching Betty direct at a favourable time, I was going off her and fell out with her over something. So we ended up as good friends. Today, she is happily married to an old friend of mine.

In the same period, now 1965, I was in the process of participating in a trip to Broadstairs. Earlier in the year my mother received an item of correspondence from Mr P or the secretary, Miss GS.

As soon as she read the contents, she told me in a friendly manner… "Michael, you're going to Broadstairs."

I felt very pleased, with no knowledge that the trip involved staying at a girls' school. Since 1963, I had always wanted to visit Broadstairs and was inspired by a selection of postcards of the resort brought back from the 1963 trip by a selection of boys participating or, taking part.

Here I was, fortunate enough participating in the trip; and, associating with female company of around my own age at the all girls' school, Bradstow.

The date, and of little relevance of the trip taking place, was on Friday, 25th June 1965. Both staff members taking the trip, had experience teaching separately, art and woodwork.

On the day of the trip the journey was smooth and for some, it was to be an exciting time. When we arrived, some of us erected a strong canvas tent catering for 12 individuals; opposite was a tennis court, the girls' school (Bradstow) and adjacent or nearby was an outdoor swimming pool where we took advantage on our first day of mixing with female company.

By the time we took to the swimming pool I felt aloof or as in the meaning 'cool and distant', observing my fellow peers striking a friendship with some female contacts.

With their conversations in 'full swing' all I could do was watch and wonder exactly what to say which is as much as I do now in certain situations. I felt lucky however avoiding any jealous feelings and getting very upset in the process.

At the school dance later that evening, I was observing these lads making headway and paying little attention to the success that these 'lucky lads' were having. Feeling undeterred from dancing with anyone, I found myself having a crush by briefly 'hanging around' and falling for a girl named Polly. Nearby was a second lad named Michael, having the same feelings for her; we were both trying to win her over so much, that it appeared a 'love triangle' was beginning.

As the evening wore on, things started 'panning out' and any fallouts over Polly were avoided. She was however, the first teenage contact that I ever had feelings for and, in recollection, I felt that the female contacts by the pool were more attractive.

With any misgivings averted with the pool contacts, I felt that falling for Polly was taking my mind off more complicated things.

At the end of the dance, I found myself having that strange 'mellow' or 'lovesick' feeling for the rest of the trip and beyond. The emotion experienced is normal for anyone starting adolescence, besides constantly thinking of a person with direct fondness.

Each night we were fortunate enough attending the dancing activities. At one of the dances, a girl called Katy was the first taking a 'shine'. As we were dancing to a slow song, she told me that I was "a nice boy". At first, I started dismissing the compliment and in the beginning I had no feelings for her or it may have saved her from getting into a spot of trouble trying to get one other girl to dance in her place.

Looking on were the staff supervising the dance and through her foolhardy actions, excluded her from the others and sent her to her room; so, following Katy's ostracisation and with limited communication skills, I was unable to try putting them to good use and mentioning her exclusion as uncalled for.

Katy must have 'felt down' for what time we had left and only cheering up when it was time for us to leave. I saw her among fellow friends, 'waving us off' from an upstairs window.

On our return to Stockgrove, I had five contacts and was writing to them all, including Polly and Katy. Where I was anticipating a reply from at least one contact, I was soon finding out that most of those participating on the trip were receiving correspondence from their girlfriends.

Feeling left out 'like a deprived child', I was feeling very upset and worthless and could only surmise or guess my circumstances surrounding this difficult period, saying to myself…

> "Where the hell did I go wrong feeling victimised like this? Was it through limited conversation with these female contacts, or, lacking experience integrating with them?"

I felt that I was being snubbed through who I was. My regular Housefather, I saw, was extremely unsympathetic; I was trying to find out whether I had any correspondence from Bradstow, and clearly saw him changing to a stroppy attitude. Unaware of my feelings or knowing how to go about the predicament that I was in, he deliberately in a very loud audible tone, said:

> "THE LAST POST WAS AT FOUR O'CLOCK. THERE'S NOTHING HERE FOR YOU!!"

With such ignorance and lacking compassion, a predicament may have arisen where I could find coping with life virtually impossible. His outburst was the last thing I needed and I found him going the right way of causing further upset to the point of needing psychiatric care.

Mr P, with any opposed opinion, may have felt compelled by sacking him for his disgraceful behaviour. Worse still, I witnessed a fellow lad crying his eyes out over the loss of a family member and looking at photographs at the same time. I saw the Housefather looking on 'stone cold'. So, making my presence felt, one must recount (or say,) "How could he sink so low?"" With no feelings or hardly any at all for anyone less fortunate than him? His attitude was…

SHAMEFUL AND COLD HEARTED!!

Following his outburst, so far I was coping, though feeling left out; unaware of an episode of fate in the 'right place at the right time' the next day.

In the mid-morning break and with the possibility of increasing my anxieties further, a staff member from House 2 appeared nearby with items of postal correspondence.

Another contact, Michael (previously mentioned) was also nearby when suddenly, among the items of correspondence, I saw a postcard addressed to a Michael Fordhead and, simultaneously, unequivocally sharp, saw Katy's name with both of us assuming that the card was meant for us.

With little social skills in mind, it was enough by speaking up for myself; arguing with ' the other' Michael that the card was mine. So 'surprising myself', I 'won the argument,' and the card was handed over. Immediately, it felt such a great relief making my presence felt, and making a very wise move at that precise moment.

Michael however felt hurt witnessing this instance and leading up to receiving that card, I had the most depressing and toughest period so far at school. The Housefather I felt, was in a 'right' dilemma who to hand the card to. So, with all due respects to his surviving family members, he deserves a mention, for appeasing my mind.

In this time period alone, I was soon finding out that at least a couple of other contacts in the same predicament experienced by myself, were wondering whether they actually had feelings for their girlfriends, or, were taking them for granted?

By taking these factors into account, I could perceive these lads feeling less sensitive with that 'don't care' attitude and leading boring lives and, inevitably in the future, leading to marital breakdown. So it goes to show the sensitivity of my nature if my predictions are right.

With the summer holidays in full swing, things were 'looking up' further when I received a second item of correspondence; this time from Cheryl whom I had no feelings for; however, we still met and visited Battersea Fun Fair.

That first date, I remember trying to win a prize for her and in conversation were talking about a younger age group attending Bradstow or as babies. Still, having no feelings or empathy and trying to pursue the relationship further, I may have increased my chances by gaining and conversing better with people.

Before taking Cheryl out, I felt unable to relate to my Bradstow associates appropriately; and how I performed may have been seen as off-putting at the start of their summer holidays.

As the coach arrived at County Hall, I met up with Polly, Katy and Cheryl. My communication skills at the time was very poor at the age I was, with little knowledge about communicating effectively. Immediately and with pen and notebook 'in hand', I began taking their contact details. There was no asking whether they were looking forward to the summer holidays, or, any holiday that they were looking forward to. Just 'straight in' like a predator catching prey without warning.

More often than not, these girls must have found themselves in an awkward situation and too polite to say anything. At the time, I remained on a steep learning curve and had much to learn. I was to find out more about this throughout my teenage years.

Meanwhile, the pupils of Bradstow were in the process of returning to school after the summer break and I felt happy seeing off two of my known contacts – both smiling and waving goodbye in the process as the coach was about to leave for the return journey. My happiness however was short-lived.

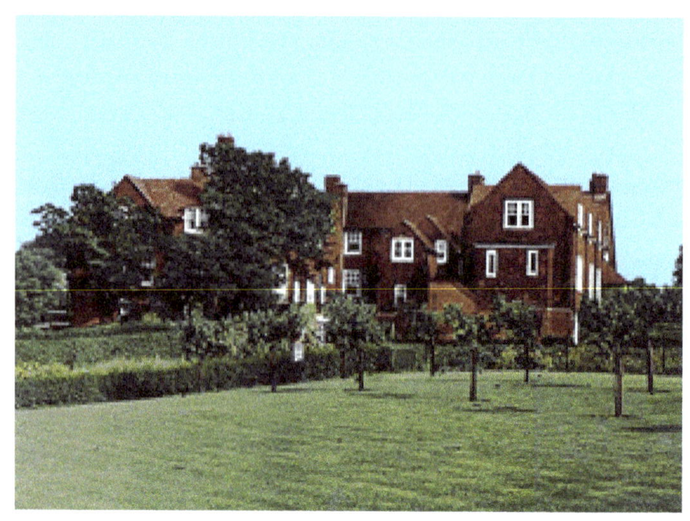

Bradstow School
The photo of this school was taken on a return visit to commemorate a previous school coach trip in the summer of 1965 I will always remember this trip for the camaraderie and the friendly atmosphere from everyone at the time. After the trip, I was unable to witness an atmosphere like this with female contacts until my regular attendance at a night club in 1980.

With the excitement dying down I got caught up with the law making my way towards Westminster Station. By composing myself inadequately, it could have seen me detained at one of the many psychiatric hospitals around at the time.

I was crossing Westminster Bridge and making my way towards the station to start the journey home. I felt that I wasn't thinking straight asking a police officer if he knew of a street, called 'Cherry Tree Lane'; a fictitious street in the film, *Mary Poppins* and one of my all-time favourite films.

He replied, "There is no Cherry Tree Lane in London."

Still besotted and locked in a fantasy world, I believed that such a street did exist in London. My fantasies about *Mary Poppins* seemed to be my downfall, with a second officer taking exception and ending up at Westminster Police Station.

I felt unconvinced with the first reply and I tried the same with another officer further along Westminster Bridge. This time, I felt unlucky with him taking hold. In the process, I started getting frustrated with him repeatedly asking the same questions. Suddenly, I tried getting away with no success. So, taking me to the nearest police station, I found myself placed among other officers in the holding area.

At some point of my stay, I thought about giving out my parents' telephone number. Soon, one of them was wondering the reason for failing to give it to the officer responsible for 'bringing me in'. At the police station, I was also told that any further attempts trying to run away would see me locked up. Appearing uncalled for making a comment on these grounds, it was as if I didn't have any rights. The Independent Police Commission was non-existent compared to today.

So far however, my family were contacted when my circumstances were explained, including my special needs and most important attending a special school for this purpose or, words to this effect, before finally being allowed to make my way home.

When leaving, I mentioned about 'no lounging around' and thought of this as a wise move through having autism. No crime however was committed on my part, and it was put down to my thoughts appearing all over the place or, as a comparison, to loose wires crossing one another.

Through experiencing things first-hand, none of the officers (so it appeared) had any idea or any personal training in autism and accounting for any neuro-diverse contact with this condition as…

Acting inappropriately or living in a fantasy world. In reality. I believe in this period that I may have been sent to a psychiatric hospital and diagnosed as plain 'mental' and, in the long term, seeking compensation later in life for any psychological damaged caused.

Since the 1990s, I have known that any individual wrongly 'locked away' can apply for compensation; in 1965 however, things were also different with plenty people 'caught up in the system' at the time of asking, 'Where is Cherry Tree Lane!?'

Now over 55 years or so 'down the line', I continue believing it normal acting out my fantasies surrounding the film, *Mary Poppins*; only however with the right people; the officer involved must have thought about my 'Cherry Tree Lane' question as a form of mockery or 'taking the rise'.

By the time I forgot about the events taking place in the holidays, we were back at school and eventually, in a better frame of mind and 'running away with myself'. Getting too excited and 'blotting out' how other people were thinking.

Unexpectedly, I had a letter from Polly and it saw me getting carried away. I knew that another Michael previously admired her. So, excited 'like a child with a brand new toy' and my excitement 'over-spilling' to him, it appeared that he was losing interest in Polly altogether.

Much is to be learnt about how to act in certain situations and every parent should follow the relevant guidelines before their child reaches puberty and adulthood to follow. Here is one example…

https://raisingchildren.net.au/autism/communicating-relationships/connecting/social-skills-for-children-with-asd

Apart from autism for example, and behaving the way I did, most of my fellow peers ended up on report during my time there. Sometimes however, a neuro-diverse autistic contact can be classed as 'naughty' while 'acting up' or on a lighter note joking around as many of us do from time to time.

Mr P however had the requisites by making a joke out of something and, in the autumn term of 1965, and on a sadder note, it saw his final term before beginning a new life in Axminster, Devon ahead of his retirement.

For a send-off, a fortnight before Mr P's departure, a special party was held for staff members and one lucky privileged lad, Kenny, who sang at the party. In class, he was very good at maths and often put on 'report' for his excellent work.

With word getting around about Mr P's retirement, some of his boys, 'deep down', were probably feeling upset and tantamount to Mrs D and Mr C in the early part of my schooling.

Mr O, the Deputy Head however, I should credit for staying the extra term for the purpose of helping the new Headmaster taking Mr P's place; he felt a true sense of 'emptiness' following his departure in 1965. We perceived him as giving us encouragement to do well in class and complimenting him, mentioning to the whole class that I had made the biggest improvement in the summer term of 1965.

Having my final say about Mr P is that he had an understanding for anyone with a disability, including autism, which is more than I can say about the new Headmaster taking his place.

CHAPTER FOUR

PART TWO

THE NEW HEADMASTER

1. A Short Introduction

At the start of the new term, many were finding out that he was very selective when it came to some of his boys choosing the trip of their choice; also depriving the wrongdoer of their privileges, such as watching television in the final recreation period, and, occasionally, using the cane for anyone doing somebody else harm. Mr P however, when making his presence felt when anyone misbehaved, abstained from resorting to the cane and took a very dim view over bullying.

When it came to Mr P's successor taking over, London was well into the swinging 60s, seen as a pleasurable time for many. The mods and rockers were still getting up to no good, with the Beatles and the Rolling Stones also going strong.

Before taking up the position as Headmaster I knew this person in May 1962 when he was teaching us in what was then, Class 2. Around this same period, Mr P was already talking about retiring and I was 'picking this up', listening to a passing conversation to my parents and a requisite to my autism.

Nearer the time, one student, Charlie, must have been the first knowing of his impending retirement. And, taking place over a game of cricket in the summer term of 1965, I too must have been the first person hearing of Mr P's successor by hearing the news from my regular Housefather.

With Christmas passing and the new term beginning on 10th January 1966, almost everyone on that first day was getting to know the Headmaster. Some of us knew him previously when he had a trial period as a teacher before advancing to his current position. As mentioned, I was one student getting to know him a few years before.

2. A New Era Begins

The first day of term saw the dawn of a new era and seeing myself, again, the first, or one of the first contacts 'picking up' on his punishing methods. Unintentionally I was doing or saying something out of place for him to say in a patronising or childish manner, that he would 'put me to bed'.

Almost immediately I got to know him better, with further incidents coming to the fore from certain contacts resenting his attitude.

This individual had a failing attitude on autism or any other hidden disabilities for that matter. I wasn't immune to his uncalled for behaviour and suffering the consequences. For some, respect appeared to be lacking and were treated like children with the punishments that he had in mind.

As he was settling into his new position, I had what was, one of many confrontations when stopping my piano practice for something I said or did; Norma, my sister, was giving free piano lessons and helping to improve my piano playing skills.

When told about his decision, I was having none of his

attitude and, defiantly, made my way into the classroom. I started playing from the music I had when suddenly and 'marching in', I was ordered to "Get out."

Still defiant I was hanging around, when he went upstairs to his living quarters, until having an outburst and shouting out loud: "I'll tell my sister about you!"

Clearly hearing my disconcertment (upset) and, approaching from his quarters, he sarcastically replied. "You can tell the Queen about me."

For the first time, I was witnessing his stubbornness and appearing that he couldn't bother with any of us apart from his wife and son, Clive, and his pet dog. I also had doubts how well he was faring with his staff, with a member leaving through the problems with his attitude.

When it was time to line up for morning activities, my regular Housefather tried finding out for himself why I was so subdued. With the answer I was giving him, he replied back. "He's on to you." I felt that at least was showing some compassion, and I was wishing it was constant.

For most of the day I was feeling very upset and being the weekend I could visit the nearest town, Leighton Buzzard, or walk round the routes on offer, giving the perfect opportunity to phone home.

At the nearest telephone kiosk, I started telling my family about the incident and in passing told them I was feeling inclined to put a chair across his head. Hearing my extreme anxiety state, they advised that it could result by landing in trouble through any serious injury caused.

So things were getting obvious that a selection of pupils in comparison, were also having issues. In his first term, one lad was expelled through a separate incident followed by a second lad a year or so later and through 'hearsay' was sent to an approved school.

So far and finding it deplorable that some of us had to 'prove the point' by using violence or threatening behaviour and talking out loud…

"It must have been making some of us think whether

he was fit running the school and showing compassion to the unfortunate with special needs? And, equally important, anyone upset by their families constantly moving? It beggars belief!"

Whatever was good to say about Stockgrove in this period was that it came with slightly relaxed discipline, or, less harshness among staff members. All along, I was usually non-violent towards my fellow pupils; I had my own problems; including one of them with a certain staff member.

When I tried fighting him, I felt that winning some self-esteem came at one of the conflicts that I had with him and arising when…

I was supposed to have been getting ready for church when caught hanging around a dormitory; as he was about to hit me, I tried hitting him back.

Before making any attempt, he came up so close that I was denied the chance; on his part, he made a very clever move. So, as quickly as it started, things were soon 'put to rest' by joining the church party and any feeling of dignity came by at least trying to 'stand up' to him.

I had at least two 'run-ins' within the space of six months or so with the next one happening when I was still in conflict with the Headmaster. This same individual, I found, had a bad habit of 'dishing up the dirt' or, bringing up any previous incident and with no exception.

In the process of taking my punishment from playing the piano, I felt better the next day to the point of messing around with one lad until caught and ended up getting a few slaps. This time, I refrained from hitting him back; all I could say was, "Watch it." This time, my pride was well and truly dented.

In the duration, I observed him 'bringing up' details that I deserved such punishment from playing the piano as one example. As the status quo stood (or was unchanged), the punishment stood with playing the piano; the only option I had, was catching up some piano practice at home.

I thought however, and in comparison to getting upset over silly little things, that he could ask us to stop 'skylarking' as the more sensible option in comparison to getting a few slaps.

One week, when Friday came, my shoes were undergoing repairs; it meant going home in my boots and, believing in perfect strangers showing me up, I chose to stay behind. By dismissing the fact that I may have been shown up by perfect strangers, a better excuse may have been feeling more comfortable wearing my shoes; in comparison, any discomfort may be felt walking around in boots for longer periods. Finding this out in recent years, online, plenty of suggestions are listed including the following…

http://www.mountainwarehouse.com/expert-advice/how-to-fit-walking-boots

In 1966, and since Stockgrove started as a school in 1950, nobody knew about certain individuals with autism disliking change. The staff member on duty, knowing of my predicament, felt inclined to lend a pair of shoes. By knowing about this any sooner, I could have used him as a fallback and taken leave as normal.

Staying behind, my parents were worried and must have contacted the school for reassurance that I was fine.

In between declining my weekend leave, Mr O the Deputy Headmaster, was standing in and I thought this a golden opportunity of catching up with some piano practice. This time, with Mr O unaware of my outstanding punishment, I decided trying my luck for a second time playing the piano but was unaware of the Headmaster's presence until he came into the classroom and confiscated my music book. This time he extended my punishment for a further two days, making in total a period of 12 days. So with the punishment taking its course, I had my book returned and allowed again, to play the piano.

3. Frustrated Over Female Contacts

With things back to normal, I felt a sense of freedom until my desperation for female company intensified with only the beginning of sheer frustration.

With no success over the Easter Holidays, I desired to return to Bradstow School, Broadstairs over the Whitsun Bank Holiday period. My request was turned down through taking part when Mr P was Headmaster.

The Headmaster's excuse I felt, was feeble and poor and going further 'beneath the surface'; whatever he was hiding, was a complete waste of time trying to obtain answers, or, the real reason for his exclusion for the trip.

Even more disgraceful came in passing conversation that three contacts who were at Broadstairs the year previously were going back. He abstained from commenting and appeared as having no feelings, offering a substituted trip to Hayling Island, Hampshire and unsurprisingly, I clearly turned down his offer.

By surmising (or guessing the real reasons) what may have taken place in the school breaks…

I was often seen standing alone at the school gates observing a crowd of females getting on and off the coach for their swimming sessions.

Sometimes, a crowd of us stood nearby, seeing them on and off the coach; when this occasion 'lent itself' I was 'blending in' and avoiding being seen as 'acting strangely'.

Unaware of my stupidity, the teachers responsible for these contacts, may have complained about my unusual behaviour. So, by fitting an accurate enough picture, my behaviour may have contributed to a refusal. However, over the years, I have been looking at the consequences by taking part in the trip and could have been spoiling things for staff and boys alike at Bradstow School and I should elaborate further on this.

With any scenario arising, I may have constantly stared at my chosen female counterpart as she was dancing with a partner. So as bad as things were, he may have been trying to save my feelings by trying to be 'cruel to be kind' and preventing anything drastic from happening. Including, the point in being so subdued, that I could easily have foreseen myself making my way to the sea front and throwing myself over the precipice (a sheer drop). So with an attempt like this failing, I too, continued seeing myself confined to a wheelchair for life.

Ringing true to any incident of this kind is the attractive Louise fitting in and imagining the upset caused seeing her pared off with somebody else.

Whatever the Headmaster was hiding, any overdue respect would have come by subtly imparting the reasons for refusing my request to go back to Broadstairs. And, giving him the respect he deserved for at least trying to mean well.

If Mr P had postponed his retirement, I could see him allowing me to return. He was that sort of character, with no intention of excluding one from an activity. His running of the school and getting the respect deserved along the way, is some achievement and admired by many school pupils. He never judged anyone through being different, in comparison to the current Headmaster making some lives a misery.

In this difficult period, I felt that while on leave in asking my father to take me to Broadstairs. I found that his van was undergoing repairs, or I could see him doing anything to make me happy. So, the only alternative I had was visiting Broadstairs by train and making my way to Bradstow from the station.

By getting to Bradstow by this method, my chances in getting the partner of my choice appeared unavoidably very slim and nothing was gained by asking my parents for the fare money to the school. So I thought about trying to 'pick up' a female contact from the street – an inadvisable move by trying to get an unknown female stranger to walk along with me. By going ahead with this method, it may have seen me 'locked up' or taken to court for harassment.

With both options failing to materialise, things appeared more wise by trying out a roller skating session at Alexandra Palace.

At the session, I observed the skaters already on the rink and was listening over the tannoy to the latest hit records. With no friends, apart from those living locally, I found myself lacking confidence talking to anyone. Now, failure in making contact, I had that terrible feeling inside and left the venue with nothing to show for it.

On the way home and failing to help the predicament that I was already in, I was passing through Finsbury Park in North London where I came across a couple near the park entrance, snogging each other. I was looking on before being seen by a friend of the couple, and found him getting stroppy (bad tempered).

Compared to offering him an apology, I chose to stay silent before continuing my journey home. He appeared obnoxious and had the opportunity dealing with things more appropriately. Sometimes however, anyone with an ASC can stare at people.

That night, I was close to tears through failing to achieve my goal. I suffered so much and was feeling insecure at the same time. My mother could only do so much trying to comfort me and now, in this 'haunting' episode, I can picture the following scenario on that fine warm sunny evening…

"With female company, I continue imagining taking advantage of the glorious weather taking place. Maybe holding hands, going for a walk in the park and snogging (or kissing) each other."

On a sad reflection, this scenario was failing to materialise. So, down on my luck, things were appearing fine for everyone else having girlfriends except for myself. I continued feeling hurt inside, thinking and writing about this all these years. I deserved better with my morale and self-esteem appearing at an all-time low.

So far, I was lucky enough coping with this difficult period or 'going under' or finding things impossible to cope with the outside world. This I felt, was no normal period and that I deserved better. I was seeking answers and getting **NONE** in return and, experiencing very sad memories.

In this same period and with the summer break upon us I was already fancying a girl living opposite and felt my frustrations getting the better of me; so, writing home, I wanted my mother's advice.

In her reply, she thought that I was too young for girlfriends. Adding that I had a better chance getting someone as I got older; already, I was failing to take any given advice and taking things the wrong way by writing a derogatory reply.

When the letter fell into the Headmaster's hands, he felt inclined to show the contents to the police before childishly tearing it up; by going that far, I could see him making a complete fool of himself. So for any respite from the troubles I was experiencing throughout the school term, things were now winding down and I was seeing more of the female contact that I was already having a soft spot for.

I found out at only 14 years of age, unknowingly, the sort of character she was. She came over rude when learning about the 'soft spot' I had through one of my friends, immediately retorting. "Well you know what he can do."

As a sensible precaution and fear of hearing any further derogatory remarks, I covered my ears before feeling hurt; with the correct social skills, I may have 'turned things around' by adding…

"That's uncalled for" and tried talking her round. Sometimes, or in many cases, a ploy of this nature usually fails and the 'injured party' must try to move on.

However, there were times when I was acting more immature than many and was easily led. One day, one of my friends jumped on the back of an ice cream van; the van was outside a block of flats and, lacking common sense, I took it upon myself to join him. So, with the van pulling away, we avoided any accidents by 'parting company' or coming off on its journey.

When we got off, I felt lucky however getting away with the driver trying to disparage and shouting out loud, "Grow up!" In the frame of mind that I was in, I may have started getting stroppy, risking getting hurt in the process, or feeling superficial through embarrassment.

Nearby, a girl called Ella, also aged around 14, was looking on with some friends, and, being nicknamed 'The Scrags' must have thought I was incompetent – a mentally deficient person or a right b*m. Through acting sensibly, I may have been on to something and had a good chance of getting something together simultaneously.

Now more the wiser and catching up with Ella for a second time in 1975, I was acting more mature; in comparison to nine years previously and finding her looking as attractive as she did in 1966.

4. Insensitive Feelings

With many events taking place six months before leaving school, I may have been better off staying at home. The Headmaster's attitude on various issues continued and I felt that this could have been doing more harm than good.

In the interim period however, I'll mention about my diary going missing and my younger sister falling very ill. So between returning to school for the autumn term, I wish to express my feelings about losing my diary and how I felt with my younger sister becoming very ill.

Since the beginning of 1965, I kept a diary for

recording daily events. Despite slow learning ability, I had fair literacy skills; my grammar however was poor as in…

Jumbled or wordy sentences

Paragraphs failing to flow or making sense

Spelling mistakes etc. (and so on)

My diary was precious until it parted company on the way home from visiting relatives in Croydon. By having the diary, I could express myself coherently by 'writing up' the day's events

On the way home, my parents and I stopped at a restaurant and thought no more about the diary staying safe in the car, or so I thought, until arriving back home. The diary parted company and no longer could I write about how I felt – expressing my anxieties, feelings, frustrations, events taking place etc. So, out of desperation and at 'first light', my parents gave me the money for the fare to go back.

As I got to the location, the diary was intact, lying in the kerb in an immaculate condition. I thought that a safer place would have been the restaurant for its safe keeping; with a heavy rainstorm taking place that night, one imagines the pages smudging beyond recognition.

Between when my diary went missing and well before, I felt self-centred around myself. Hardly feeling sorry for anyone and in most cases, lacking empathy until late September.

A common cold virus was going around and, as before, a variety of illnesses can arise including severe bronchitis, laryngitis in adults or croup in the very young.

Barbara, my younger sister, aged 3, had croup. An infection of the throat making it hard to breathe and understandably it caused her to become very restless ahead of the paramedics taking her to hospital.

On the way to the hospital she was put on oxygen

to help her breathe, and on arrival put straight into a steamed incubator to loosen the phlegm obstructing her airways.

In my parents' absence, Norma and I had been taking care of our grandmother who also felt unwell and was recuperating with us before she was well enough to go home. Josephine however was a couple of years older than Barbara, but may have been too young to know of Barbara's illness. So, learning more about the disease, the link below has further information about its symptoms:

http://www.nhs.uk/Conditions/Croup/Pages/Complications.aspx

When my parents returned from the hospital later in the day, I found the atmosphere very subdued. In recollection and recounting, "I have **NEVER** witnessed an atmosphere like this before." Also, I cannot forget two songs that were around at the time:

'All strung out.'	Nino Tempo and April Stevens
'Cherish.'	The Association

Today, I find it uncomfortable listening to these songs. Fortunately however, Barbara made a full recovery and my family and I had many happy years together until her passing in 2001.

When it was time to return to school, the new term had hardly started when I fell ill myself with a bad cold and asthma to follow and I tried treating myself by buying some tablets in town. As soon as starting them, my condition was taken less seriously by the Headmaster advising that treating myself would see me getting some of his treatment.

Taken aback, it appeared that he could 'talk down' to whoever he pleased, making him an obnoxious and ignorant character. He failed to realise the seriousness of asthma interfering with one's breathing and the risk of death in a very severe attack.

When getting to see the school doctor, I was asked if I had asthma since childhood; by 'filling him in' about the condition, I was put on tablets to take morning and night.

The Headmaster's very poor popularity with many fall-outs by fellow pupils, I felt that he was putting the unlucky few into 'bad light' and also undermining many with his punishing regimes and making many feel inferior.

The discipline criteria was also lacking, resulting in an element of teasing in the school breaks. Throwing stones and being looked on as a 'soft touch'. Autism however meant nothing to my fellow students. Let alone its meaning and the effects on each individual.

When the minority started throwing stones, I used a dustbin lid on the odd occasion for protection; in a separate incident, I found myself in an embarrassing position and ordered inside the school building by a school teacher.

As a Martial Arts expert in Judo, his order I felt, was unnecessary and in place he should have been ordering the perpetrators to stop or return to their classes. By using his authority I felt, would impart the respect from anyone with more understanding towards somebody less fortunate.

Later, I remember confronting one individual where, I must have ended up either pushing or hitting him for his wrongdoing; he turned out to be a 'fine friend' until 'easily led' with the 'stone throwing' incidents.

In addition to the way I was, there were times when I acted strangely including constantly putting my radio to my ear and listening to any song taking my liking; things too, were the same outside the school surroundings, and occasionally I was 'caught out' by the 'locals' witnessing my strange behaviour.

Very often and apart from the friends I already had, I saw myself as an 'oddball'; hardly mixing with anyone and choosing to be alone. Now, and so far, the only pupil feeling victimised, or so it appeared. Another lad,

Charlie, a new boy, eventually started having the 'same treatment' through his disability.

Witnessing the teasing with him, "I wished, saying to myself that I could have tried helping him by trying to get these so-called kids to back off and leave him alone;" by accomplishing this, I believe that perhaps I may have gained back some of my 'lost pride'.

Charlie however, and as ironic as it gets, chose a career in the army which may have 'toughened' him up, or, helped him learn to deal better with past teasing incidents.

Coinciding with things, I was however in the process of leaving school and before this I had the privilege of taking charge of a table serving five lads until these lads started 'playing up' and being called a 'Jew Boy'. A name I had to put up with throughout my time until leaving in 1967.

Unable to redress any teasing, the Headmaster had to intervene by putting somebody else in charge; by challenging him, he tried meaning well. Adding that it was far short of any punishment and that this lad should be put in charge.

With three weeks to go before leaving, I was taking his decision well. A gastric flu epidemic was going around in the early part of 1967; with no exception, I ended up violently sick.

In a letter to my family, I was mentioning about my recent illness before he got hold of the letter and taking exception to the contents, tore it up. I was clearly seeing him insinuating or assuming that I was bolting my food and insisting on handing over any sweet-related items from my weekly parcels – including biscuits, chocolate or, stopping my piano sessions for two weeks.

By now, I was perceiving him as having no time for anyone's feelings. More of an attitude problem and many must have been having doubts about his position as Headmaster. By expressing my honest opinion and thinking to myself…

"I had doubts about his mentality running the school and for some making their lives a misery." With the outside authorities finding out his methods and unable to run the school efficiently, that somebody else may have taken over in the role of Headmaster. Just anyone with an understanding towards us.

I felt in this period with many falling sick with this bug, that I was again, a few weeks away from leaving school and starting a new life.

5. The Youth Club

The final section in this chapter on my school days is about my experiences at this club which existed in Leighton Buzzard; the club no longer exists through catching fire and razed to the ground by arsonists.

In the club's heyday, it was very popular with a few lads from Stockgrove, joining up in the summer term of 1966; compared to Bradstow in Broadstairs, an all girls' school. The club contained a mixed element of neuro-typical teenage boys and girls attending and I soon became part of it.

Getting to the club was easy enough and only a 30-minutes' cycle ride away and, helping things further, was the friendliness of the current members as I was getting known. A member cracked a joke at the expense of his mate snogging his girlfriend; I was checking the time on my watch when he joked, "Are you timing it?" With the right attitude on his part, I appeared auspicious enough avoiding any 'flack' this time round.

For any newcomer, some of us had to 'blend in' and feel accepted. I soon found myself part of the club with my autism, proving to be no problem. As an 'extra bonus' it would have been good getting off with a gorgeous-looking blonde girl that I had the 'hots' for.

My fellow peers however must have felt more shy than myself. I felt lucky that seeing this blonde on the one occasion, prevented a 'full blown' crush from materialising. I had to make do with someone far less attractive – a contact named Hilary when she was taking a 'shine'. I felt the opposite with hardly any feelings for her and that I had to end the friendship that we had and we both stopped writing. By then, I had left school.

By taking account anyone lucky enough pairing off with a partner was a contact named Kenneth. He was no trouble to anyone and I cannot understand him getting a severe beating off his regular Housefather in the early part of his schooling.

With Kenneth's success and as a normal emotion, I was feeling jealous of his female associate as they held hands. Things however would have been much worse, by 'bonding' with the blonde contact that I was liking a few months before. At the same time as Kenneth's success were some 'great pretenders', bragging about getting off with their chosen female counterpart.

Through having a clearer mind many years later, I felt that I was taking things far too seriously. Not knowing whether my fellow peers or lads were taking advantage, or trying to have a sick joke at my expense, then, getting upset in the process.

Things however turned out false and I felt so relieved. Some of my former club associates may have had marital breakdowns and/or have failed keeping long-lasting friendships.

With the time getting near to leaving school, I was in the process of leaving and starting out in tailoring. So ahead of getting to my chosen career and the jobs I had in between, I am taking the opportunity by summing up my stay at the school.

In the preceding sections of this chapter on my school days, my experiences are a sad reflection, taking into account anyone else under the same circumstances. Including…

The frustrations of living with autism and communicating ineffectively, my nerves plainly holding me back and lacking in confidence.

CHAPTER FIVE

FIRST TASTES OF EMPLOYMENT

1. First Jobs

Leading on to leaving school, I have decided to break things down by mentioning my experiences working for various organisations. I shall be returning to events taking place in my younger years, once making my experience known with these organisations.

Breaking things down, I feel, would give this book more of a flavour and as an alternative to integrating events into chronological order as my life went on.

My first taste of work experience came as far back as April 1966. It was the Easter holidays and 'as good a time as any' for trying something new.

My father was previously in the tailoring trade and suggested that I 'follow in his footsteps'; he knew the managers running a firm at Oxford Circus. I worked for them in this time period and learnt to use a thimble – a useful 'tool' when it came to repairing garments or sewing buttons on items of clothing.

In between working at another tailoring firm, my second 'taster' of work came in September working briefly for the PDSA (People's Dispensary for Sick Animals). The duties were, collecting various clothing items, bric-a-brac etc. from various institutes and organisations and bringing them back to the depot.

Anything of intrinsic or sentimental value was sold on and the money made for helping sick or injured animals. I, however, lasted the day and left through the teasing by fellow teenage employees taking unfavourable advantage of my gentle side or, who I was. In between the journeys to the various destination, I constantly asked them to leave me alone.

As we got to South London, we stopped at a South London girls' school. 'Out of the blue' one of the lads spat at the girls for no-good reason and it was clear to see that he had problems. The bewildered individuals were shocked and thinking to themselves how disgusting he was. Through reproaching this individual, I may have seen repercussions taking place but I chose to stay quiet to prevent this from happening.

In between arriving back, the teasing continued and further problems arose back at the depot where I had a book thrown at me. Whatever I was meant to have said or done remained unjust by the individual responsible. I felt undermined and unable to 'stand up' to them without the risk of getting hurt; so using my instincts, I had the common sense leaving the PDSA and having no further association with these individuals.

Between starting the school term and leaving in March 1967, I had a break trying out any further jobs. Over Christmas 1966, my father arranged an interview at another tailoring firm. The firm was Simpsons in Stoke Newington, Hackney where I met the Director in charge of the Company.

The interview was very formal and compared to an interviewer asking loads of questions. I soon found out about my success, with the position reserved following the Easter holidays (1967). So, starting work, I had no worries and felt relatively calm and hoping that I could make a career out of tailoring.

In 1967, the 'state of play' with finding work appeared less forthcoming by a 'slump' in the job market. When I started, I found the learning process stressful until, in a day or so, something 'clicked'. Finding at last, I could machine-stich. So, getting the basics, I tried matching the various patterns and learning to stitch in a straight line. I was finding this very hard and so, unsuccessfully trying to master this skill, I was soon dismissed.

Leading up to this, I was sent to see the Line Manager's boss for messing around and failing to take the tasks accomplished, seriously enough, or, through poor performance.

At the meeting, I found him patronising enough and near enough succeeding in disparaging my self-worth and interjecting that my fellow contacts were progressing to making items of clothing, including shirts, trousers etc.

Hearing what he had to say, I mentioned some contacts having a 'head start' at school, learning to sew and seeing them proficient by using a sewing machine. With such ignorance and making a good job keeping his composure, I saw his weak side, dismissing my points and believing that none of his employees had any training before coming into the job.

He too, thought himself clever. 'Putting me down' further, while back in the workplace and making a remark about my work and retorting sarcastically…

"Nice isn't it?" When, clearly, the practice pieces accomplished were substandard.

Witnessing such ignorance, he was seen as failing and going 'beneath the surface' and, having no time finding out my 'weak points' in certain areas. The company had more of an interest getting as much work out of their employees as possible and having no time for slow learners or anyone with an autistic impairment.

The line manager, I thought, was as bad when I told her outright that I was 'doing my best'.

Her reply was. "You are not paid to do your best. You are here to work."

With such ignorance, she failed finding out…

The reasons for my slow performance and finding it hard machining straight with the practice samples and also matching the clothing patterns.

With things moving on – a Work's Tribunal is one option that an employee can turn to for any employer or employees acting inappropriately.

In 1967, the word 'Autism' meant very little with less help out there compared to today; through this, I had to leave the job. So I was called to the Director's office where, my line manager, director and a family member were present. With a decision given about my dismissal, I parted on friendly terms ahead of two more unsuccessful attempts trying to 'break into' the tailoring trade.

2. First Steady Job –The Painting Trade

No autistic work-related agencies existed until the 1990s; when they did exist, the candidate could assign a Support Worker supporting him or her in the work place.

Before autism was more established, I was having to 'fend' for myself. I tried 'mastering' the tailoring trade with my last attempt coming at the beginning of May 1967 working for a firm, 'Brummels'. I was only there for the day when I was asked to leave by their line manager, through unsuccessfully trying to keep to a timescale.

With no understanding about autism, anyone can be 'under the impression' that very few firms made any allowances for slow learners. This however, has changed with any employer compelled to make changes for anyone with a disability, whatever form and making adjustments accordingly.

By filling in my family about losing my job, I decided on taking up a career in the painting trade. In between this period before entering the trade, I was working at a zip factory and, to follow, a warehouse packing handbags.

Ahead of the interview, I attended evening classes in woodwork at college and mentioned this when the interview took place for the painting and decorating position at Hackney Town Hall. I felt that through college breaking up, that the interview was bad timing.

As the interview was taking place, the interviewer asked whether I was still attending an evening class in woodwork. Already, the college had 'broken up' and unknowingly I was 'side-tracked' when asked by the interviewer…

"So you have been attending an evening class in woodwork. Are you still attending?" My reply was, "No, I don't do it any more."

Now more the wiser, I feel that I could have turned things around by increasing my chances working for Hackney and should have turned things round by articulating…

"Yes, I have been attending an evening class in woodwork. Before classes start in September, I will find out whether a class specifically on painting and decorating exists. That way, I can gain the additional knowledge required where, I can put these skills to good use while working for you."

Today any employer knowing beforehand that a candidate has autism, the key worker can go about informing the employer ahead of any interview. The NAS website covers this well.

By failing the interview with Hackney Council, I was soon successful when a vacancy for my chosen position arose at Islington Council and I felt compelled 'staying focussed' throughout.

At the interview, both my parents were present with the interviewer, the Building Works Manager; as it progressed, I was given a selection of mathematical-related questions and asking whether I needed any paper to write down the answers. I replied, "No, it's fine, I can work things out."

By getting some, or, all the answers right, it appeared inevitable, that by creating such a good impression, that I was successful.

With the interview over, I soon saw this as an achievement and getting away from the monotony working in dead-end jobs, or, jobs consisting of a poor salary. Now with a proper job, my rate of pay was to be much higher compared to vacancies with no future.

On the first day, I made my way to the depot having been given an address; I was hoping that before arriving at a flat in the Holloway area that it was to be the start in learning the trade. It became a misconception.

On arrival, I was met by a contact with 40 years' worth of experience behind him and I was left hanging around doing nothing; I felt under the impression that his only concern was to carry on working and I was looked on as a 'second class citizen'.

Soon, I was getting so fed up that I started complaining about my boredom; failing to show any concern, I found him unfriendly and disrespectful and choosing to talk about his time duration in the painting trade.

I felt that by being made to feel welcome, that the chances were there by learning more about me and implying that I was only staying with him for a short time duration; so, filling in time, I could have been tidying up the flat, or trying some painting.

Feeling that I wasn't listened to, I chose to leave the flat, calling my parents from a nearby telephone box and in passing said that I wanted to come home before being advised to 'sit it out' longer ahead of the foreman making his presence. So, making my way back to the flat, the foreman showed an address of a vacant property nearby.

When getting to the property, I was introduced to a contact hoping to sustain his role by learning the trade of painting and decorating. So, settling in, my first task was painting window frames in green paint and accomplishing other tasks simultaneously. Laughing and 'joking around' with my contact or, to a finer point, a mate happy going along with my childish attitude until things started turning sour.

At the next property, I was doing or saying something out of turn and specifically, remembering this day well; the previous day, I was upset over Radio London, a former offshore pirate station closing down for good. Through failing to focus properly, my mate threw a paint brush which could have seen me rebelling and leading to dismissal through misconduct.

With my pride taking a 'knock back', my mother was seeing herself through trying to prevent any further incidents, and gave a letter for my mate to show more understanding. I was with him for a further three weeks until placed with somebody stricter.

3. The New Contact

Two months on from starting the job, I was placed with a new but stricter mate with no idea on autism and resulting in occasional fall outs.

My first inkling or suspicions came when I tried getting off early to meet a girlfriend. Seeing his true character as authoritarian and patronising came when asking, "Where do you think you're going?"

At 16 and with the frustrations of adolescence, I was feeling that I was having enough problems of my own; the way he was treated in his younger days, may have been 'rubbing off' when he was learning the trade, he was having his 'a**e kicked' whenever his work fell to an unacceptable standard.

As if things weren't bad enough, I was also putting up with one of his associates, appearing as bad while working under him for a short period. Shouting through finding it hard trying to get my work to an acceptable performance and throwing a paintbrush on the floor.

Feeling that I could do more, I may have ended up throwing a tin of paint over him and risked getting hurt. Weighing things up, I was finding this associate pleasant enough with his jokes and laughing in the process.

My regular mate was showing his displeasure and sometimes, I was walking off the job and I continue recalling one classic example…

One day, and failing to think straight, I unintentionally left the windows open for the paint to dry in the ground-floor flat and left to do some shopping. On my return, I barely walked through the door when I got pushed. Taking exception to his actions, I felt determined against putting up with his behaviour any further and walked off the job.

Trying to 'kill time', I cycled around the locality before making my way home and informing my parents about the incident and finding them unsympathetic. With very little understanding about the circumstances involved, they may have been thinking to themselves that working under a 'firm' character, would help with my learning.

I had a second opinion, thinking to myself…

"How can things follow when 'undermining me?'; including. "You never learn. Do you?" "Why do I keep rucking you?" And, "Don't catch yourself alight," when too slow on the job. I had to also put up with his regular 'put downs' when I wasn't doing the job to his liking and this wasn't all.

When trying to look superior in front of fellow painters, he would say…

> "I am trying to make him stand on his own two feet."
>
> "You're the least important man on the firm."

…and "A man who doesn't have any pride in his appearance has no pride in his work," referring to my dirty overalls when stripping wallpaper – a remark which, I believe, is as ignorant as it can get as well as showing off and often gloating over the management being less than impressed with my work performance.

So far, his remarks were 'out of character' and clearly anyone could have seen him as a 'total idiot' and a couple of times, I was telling him that I could get along better with other painters. Clearly showing his displeasure, he retorted, "Am I too strict then?"

With such ignorance as before, it appeared that none of his fellow painters dared speak up for me, through the risk of any consequences that they may have faced.

I was hardly learning and placed with the wrong type of people. Including the Building Work's Manager who, also, took a dim view of my behaviour and I was summoned to him by the foreman following the first incident – leaving the windows open to dry and walking off the job following my mate's bullying tactics.

A Union however existed but I felt that they were there only for settling disputes on a wider scale, including pay and working conditions; or I could have taken the easy way out – leaving the job and working for an outside firm.

At only 18 at the time when these various incidents were arising, my mate went sick, meaning one thing – a break from his undermining and patronising behaviour; this was the break needed for some recess or 'time-out'.

When returning from sick leave through a bad back, no further incidents arose until something happened with him acting bossy and articulating abruptly through doing or saying something to his disliking…

"I want you to wash those coves!" (The concave surface in place of skirting boards.)

Answering back, I mentioned that they didn't need doing. Suddenly, and taking hold, he started 'shaking me like a rat'. As he was finishing, I retorted, "I will not be walked over" and intended sitting outside the flat when the foreman arrived, seeing for himself the altercation unfolding.

In his presence, he was making it clear that he didn't want me back. So, collecting my tools, it was recommended that I accompany the foreman to the depot.

On the way down, I found myself shaking inside. My mate's actions were totally unnecessary, he was a total bully and this time, 'Behaving like a real total idiot' or, going one better, a stupid 'nutter' seeing myself as a failure with this type of a mate. His patience I also felt, was limited and often undermining for no apparent reason.

At the depot I stayed until the end of the working day and, filling in time performing odd jobs. Including painting doors ready to go on site and, ahead of going with somebody else happy taking a supervising role. Hearing about the events unfolding with my mate, I thought that at least he could have sympathised in place of showing any disappointment.

Ben however, another painter, had already witnessed past episodes of humiliation and, having the right attitude, I was finding him very kind and sincere believing that if he could put my mate 'in his place', then he would have been the one standing up for me.

With such a sincere person, I believe that I should have worked for him for his true and understanding attitude, at the same time learning the trade off him and putting my mate to shame in the process.

Both my parents once more took a dim view, with no realisation about his humiliation and undermining when trying to learn a proper trade; my mother also went on to say that he was a 'smashing bloke'. My parents however never got to know what he was really like, and trying to get through to them may have been a waste of time.

On the lighter side of things, they perceived me as a slow learner or, labelled as ESN (Educationally Sub Normal). Today, this is classed as a Specific Learning Difference which sounds much better.

My mate I thought, failed by 'picking up' on these impairments and that I went to a special school; his reply was…

"Well, that's why I am so tolerant."

By acting on his comment, I could have told him about my previous bad experiences. Including…

- A virtual outcast when I was much younger with hardly any friends.
- The troubles encountered trying to act the same as my school peers.
- Taken to Westminster Police Station by a Police Officer believing that I was 'taking the rise' by asking whether he knew of a 'Cherry Tree Lane'; I was already near Big Ben and the Houses of Parliament at the time and a fair distance from any residential streets.
- Teased at school through 'being who I was'.

And so on…

These brief 'key factors', and with my family writing a letter, may have seen him having a better understanding and taking into account my impairments and making him see sense.

So far, and hardly able to think for myself by making things better, I had to 'parry' his ignorant remarks making me feel undermined and besides his 'put downs' and hardly getting anywhere learning a decent trade off him.

Up to now, his behaviour was 'absolutely disgraceful' along with the staff above him responsible for 'siding' along with him.

In the same period, the painter I was with, saw a break from this 'patronising' individual and I was feeling much happier with him playing a role and at least, learning a trade. As the status quo stood however, I could no longer stay with him through 'bodging' or failing to do the job properly.

With one thing in mind, and to my displeasure, the foreman was suggesting a 'very' foolhardy act – recommending a return to the contact that I was having trouble with. In between the fall outs I had, I found things more peaceful and relaxed in the company of other painters and now the foreman was upsetting the status quo. The latter meaning 'unchanged'.

In between this period, the Christmas period was getting near with the Council adjourning for the break; with things back to normal. I felt that I had to end up 'grinning and bearing' the thought of returning to my mate.

Finally going back to him, the first thing I noticed was seeing him showing some respect and anticipating learning the art of paper-hanging; a skill I was yet to learn. His problem came when finding fault with my work and failing on keeping his promise. So, I had to learn myself or leave the trade entirely through feeling reluctant doing painting alone.

By thinking on his decision with him doing a 'U' turn, that things might have worked in my favour by…

Asking that I should be taught to learn to hang paper and gaining the respect from everyone and to stop finding fault with my work.

With this ploy appearing a hopeless cause, I could have walked off the job and gone sick.

By tolerating whatever was coming, I continued working under him, unaware that by the summer period things were ending working with this 'so-called' mate.

When the end came, I was finishing my apprenticeship at college where, even there, my fellow students were teasing me until getting advice from family on how to act more sensibly with them. Until then the teasing continued before eventually, stopping together.

In this period, I was working in the depot and in between 'venturing' out on various jobs under a supervisor and, a brief spell working alone in various flats.

At last, this brief spell was a start to self-teaching

myself the methods in paper hanging. A role that my so-called mate should have carried out in comparison to painting only. Throughout much of 1971 however, the intermittent jobs continued including painting flower pots and warning signs warning drivers of an oncoming bend, as examples.

I felt however that with the trend of working in empty properties that I could gain extra experience in paper hanging, simultaneously preventing any grievances with the foreman in charge working at the depot.

By falling out, I felt that things could have been resolved and prevented also, from seeing the Works Manager, in less formal terms 'the Governor'; at first, I was refusing to co-operate by going in front of him.

As the foreman continued the pressure, I found the Works Manager acting stroppy and that I was only half a painter – implying that my work was sub-standard. With such insulting tactics, I felt that I could have had a 'right go' at him and risk putting my employment into jeopardy or, a good chance of getting sacked.

At this time, much stigma came about relating to people with autism; consequently, I and many others on the spectrum, took much 'flack'. Normally, most neuro-diverse contacts show no signs of any violence or, things may have been different with the perpetrator put in his rightful place. Things however were about to improve.

Before Christmas I was soon back working in void properties and to my delight and, in time for Christmas, was granted the privilege of taking part in a bonus scheme. At last, I saw myself learning a proper trade in comparison to accomplishing menial tasks.

The recommendation prevented any further fallouts with the foreman and I felt happier between 1972 and 1980; taking advantage of earning extra money by getting as much work done in the shortest possible time.

4. Trying For Promotion

The first instance when I started losing pride came as far back as 1976 when I tried gaining promotion for the Supervisory Craftsman position; a position supervising painters.

Before the interview, I had no idea about filling out an application form successfully. I was compiling the form as…

> **Qualifications**
> 'Top of the class in maths' in comparison to:
> Maths A Level
> English O Level
>
> City and Guilds – Painting and Decorating, etc.

Ironically, I was successful enough getting an interview; at which the person in charge started asking whether I had any questions; very foolishly and unconsciously, I asked whether I needed a briefcase for the job.

Through lacking this knowledge, I felt undermined by the lucky candidate securing the position; much to my surprise however and, in time, he gave up the position through the stress involved.

On hearing this, perhaps it may have been unwise applying for the Supervisory Craftsman position at the time. A suitable position may have arisen with one exception.

Between late 1977 to 1979, I had frequent episodes of sick leave and seeing the firm's doctors. This was unknowingly putting my promotion prospects in jeopardy. I have asthma and in between bad episodes, I was often taking sick leave.

I found these attacks more frequent after being admitted to hospital with severe breathing difficulties. Almost coinciding in this period alone, there were no voids or empty properties. Only working outside in the freezing cold and taking extra sick leave as a precaution.

When my health improved, I tried applying for a foreman's position and through taking too much time off sick, I was denied an interview; my demands were ignored and I felt victimised through no fault of my own. In the late 1970s, any discrimination in age, gender, disability etc., hardly saw any victim of circumstance ever standing a chance in a career change.

In this period, trying for promotion on the Council appeared a waste of time and I chose trying to find alternate employment in an office-related environment through the Employment Exchange.

On my arrival, I found the vacancies offering less than a painter and decorator; others required qualifications. All I wanted was for the elimination of 'red tape' with these vacancies and a trial period in its place. This method is better than undergoing an interview and in some jobs, passing the Short Answer Test before the interview; in the past, I failed and ever since I've felt deterred from taking further tests of this kind.

With the advertised vacancies a lost cause, I made an appointment to see the Employment Advisor to try finding out whether I could work at something else. He was very unhelpful by failing to find…

> The length of time spent in the Painting Trade.
>
> Any previous jobs before working for the Council.
>
> Any disabilities and a possible trial period with a respectable and understanding employer.

His negative views came when 'skimming the surface' and advising that I needed to attend evening classes before any respected employer would think of 'looking at me'. My rights were totally disregarded. I felt betrayed and denied a chance in the job market; at least trying to work round the 'qualification' issue, I may have been offered a trial period in my chosen career, working in an office-related environment.

Today, we have this cliché about equal opportunities, where one must accomplish the following…

> Completing an application form and seeking help filling it in.
>
> The Interview: This is where many Neuro Diverse individuals 'fall down'.

With the respect lacking, I could have addressed my complaints to the Manager. Perhaps then, if I could have 'spoken up for myself', then he/she may have acted on my behalf.

Leaving the Employment Exchange, I continued feeling bitter and undermined and wish to elaborate further on this:

Early in 1979, three of my fellow painters were promoted to the Foreman position. In protest, I could have taken sick leave until offered alternate employment such as a clerical position; another alternative is deliberately losing the Council money by ignoring their bonus scheme and working slow.

In the course of protesting I may have been summoned to see the Work's Manager; by taking a sympathetic view, he may have helped with any alternate employment position suited for my needs.

So, I am making **NO** apologies by making my presence felt with the Council and the Employment Advisor. The way I was treated is **ABSOLUTELY DISGRACEFUL**. I was treated like s**t following the three individuals promoted to Foreman.

With things bad enough, another Foreman applied to work for the Council, finding while working under him further 'dented pride' to come.

5. Champion Pride Taker

I got to know this individual in 1980 and saw him as the authoritarian type. I also saw him as undermining and taking away one's pride.

At first glance, he seemed reasonable enough and thought no more of him until finding fault with my work. I tried taking advantage of the bonus scheme by giving the doors and fittings one coat of paint to save time.

To him, he appeared unhappy with my ploy and called for his superintendent. I thought this a 'sick joke' and I had a right go at him on his return. As I started calming down, his words were, "It's good to have a go." This meant nothing and thought that he was wasting the superintendent's time by visiting me.

While unable to comprehend him sinking so low, I soon started getting to know his true character as threatening at times to anyone weaker than him and his alleged brothers backing him up when finding himself in trouble. In generalising this, I now believe that through his cowardice, that he was putting on a front.

At the time, I was 29 years of age with hardly any confidence trying to 'stand up to him'. This rang true when insinuating or threatening to put me with some undesirable, all through what he thought of as poor work performance on my part and working too slow in the process. I could have tried undermining him by recounting, "You are so ignorant that you ought to be ashamed of yourself." Then he may have turned nasty and perhaps so insulting, that I may have felt more humiliated and speechless in the process.

With his 'put down', he placed me with someone released from prison for robbery. This shady character I was to find false, and I saw myself a victim of a con.

His first ploy came on the pretence of losing his wages and, in an irate state, asked if I could lend him any money to tied over. Being the fool I was, I agreed. In my absence, the foreman called and spoke about docking my time. Hearing this, the guy told him to back off. I could clearly see the foreman appearing timid, while informing quietly about docking my pay by half an hour. So whatever his ploy was about having as many as six brothers, it appeared he was 'putting on a front' and making a bad job of things in the process.

Following things through, I was conned a second time when asked if I desired going into business with him; he pretended that the extra money was for plant and materials to get started. Continuing to be so naive, I had so far lost in total £100 and could have lost more on another occasion with three other associates visiting the flat.

In the process, one of them presented me with a £60 cheque and asked me to cash it at the bank; knowing full well that the cheque was going to 'bounce', I refused to co-operate and ended getting smacked in the mouth by the guy I was working with; he perceived me as betraying his father whose cheque it was.

At the earliest opportunity with his associates leaving and remaining alone in the flat, I gathered my tools and belongings, made my way to the depot and reported the incident to the superintendent.

Returning to the depot Monday morning, I found out that the guy had absconded ahead of getting a visit from the foreman telling him, "I want you to come with me. I am not leaving until you do."

If true, then I could see him 'taking my side'; as a safety precaution however, I reciprocated that I should be placed elsewhere and out of harm's way with the prospect of his associates returning.

So with £100 down, things quietened down at work until one day, I started seeing the foreman's true character through getting upset over a silly little thing.

A fellow painter associate was working in the same block of flats where I was placed. In passing conversation,

I asked what he thought of the foreman. With my remark 'getting back', he came over in a threatening manner as in "Now, I want you to get the paint spots off the floor." In the process, I thought that I was about to get hit following my remark; I was very fortunate getting away with nothing more than his patronising ways.

Feeling resentful, I informed my family, that I would eventually end up 'smacking him in the mouth' if he carried on continually patronising me. They offered no sympathy, parrying my resentment at the same time. Now the pinnacle of my pride was dented further. I felt too scared to talk, with the whole issue being most humiliating.

By now, I started perceiving him as a troublemaker while at the depot picking up some items to take back to the flat. In front of his fellow staff members, he recounted that one of the painters that I was working alongside with, earned my bonus for me.

His working partner observing his behaviour, advised that I should speak up more; by speaking up more, I would be asking him to stop his patronising ways in front of everyone. So, a good point comes by 'trying on' his behaviour outside work and in a social situation and getting hurt in the process. The same difference can also arise by bragging that he had six brothers.

As his behaviour was getting too much I was in the 'throws' of taking sick leave. This may have been a dilemma, losing my temper and risking losing my job.

Returning from sick leave, I found him very pleasant until my accident taking building plant, paint, etc., down a flight of stairs where, I felt my back go; little knowing that the accident was developing itself into severe Sciatica, I carried on working.

In this short space of time or coinciding, I observed him reverting back to his old ways when talking about my accident and unbelievably coming out with a derogatory remark…

"No one cares about how you feel."

Clearly, he was lacking in intelligence and unaware of the consequences arising out of my accident. As well as his untoward behaviour, I perceived him as an embarrassment whenever he spoke about sex. And, perceiving seeing my 'arse' going up and down and on one occasion, trying to 'touch me up' with his hand on my leg and over-praising whenever I worked well.

On the opposite side of things, he was often annoyed whenever I was working too slowly. In narrating the bad things about him, came one exception when he had a right showing any discontent.

I was working at an occupied property when I started having a 'mental block'. By failing to think straight, I unintentionally failed to cover the carpet and furniture properly which resulted in ceiling soft white falling on the exposed areas.

On the occupant's return, I was finding myself in 'deep' trouble when she called the depot. My foreman started making his presence and I got a right b*****g, with him 'going over the top' and undermining at the same time. This time in front of the apprentice taking my place and acting sarcastically flamboyant. Perceiving too that he was getting the *Daily Mirror* involved.

By trying to 'get one over' him, I could have seen him making a 'right fool' out of himself by going to a national newspaper and being made a 'complete laughing stock'.

In comparison to the superintendent arriving, I saw him taking a dim view and feeling disappointed at the same time. This felt reasonable and I felt helpless with the situation that I was in.

As I was leaving, the younger guy was 'filling in' that through my 'slip up', 'he' (the foreman) started 'letting it out' with my fellow painters, or, bossing them around. So, saying to myself: "It goes to show, the kind of a man he was."

When I had to leave, I went to a rundown occupied property. I was getting known by the occupier, who, with his help, I wrote a letter of an apology to the previous occupier. Paddy, the owner of the property, was sympathetic by what happened.

Under the circumstances, writing that letter was the right thing to do and soon found out that cleaning the furniture came close to £100. In time and taking my punishment working in a couple of substandard properties, I was soon allowed to work back in a better property environments.

Previously, I had known his ways of punishing individuals by…

'Placing those in the dirtiest, rundown properties that he could find.'

When things were back to normal, everything as usual was fine until a show of protest in 1981 at a vacant flat near Upper Street.

At the flat, the foreman made sure by undermining further and that I would be in trouble by failing to work more quickly. When that failed, he started acting in a 'rather' bolshy way.

"Now, I want you to earn a bonus."

The way he was coming across, I started asking whether he intended informing the Superintendent. His reply was that he would, where interjecting that I was not keen in that earning any bonus may have been the better option or, deliberately biding my time to finish the job.

With his undermining tactics, I was feeling very resentful once more. With so much anger, my intentions were to cycle to the depot on Monday morning and with any 'bottle' whack him with bicycle chain with the lock attached to the end; it may have resulted in losing my job and/or being sent to prison. However, it could have served a purpose, with him thinking twice about humiliating or patronising anyone else or ending up in real danger by 'trying it on' with the wrong people. So, before coming back to events taking place, I noticed something in his possession capable of harming anyone upsetting him.

On the odd occasion I saw that he had a gun; so, any intention of trying to harm him I could end up seeing myself crippled or, shot dead; as a grim reality needing that gun for protection, and, showing the type of character that he was.

Through coming from a decent and respectable family that I should go as far as saying…

“I was **NEVER** brought up as a fighter, or the type meddling with danger in the criminal world.”

So far and to an autistic person the events unfolding before my ‘very’ eyes may have been frightening. So, no matter what consequences I may face in the future, I feel that it takes much encouragement and/or bravery writing about the predicament I was met with by working for the Council. Today, I continue finding the way that he was performing so surreal and unbelievable.

So perhaps by aborting my first plan by ‘whacking’ him with my bicycle chain, I came up with something better and chose to lock myself in the flat. Believing that he would stop any ‘slagging off’ or, ‘running down’ my pride, I knew this time that he was going too far. I knew previously of a painter who tried the same thing, and that it appeared to work. So I followed suit by placing the key in the lock, stopping him from entering with the spare key he had.

Finding himself unable to gain access, his exact words were, “Open this door. You’re stopping me from getting into the flat.” By flatly refusing, I felt that I was beginning to make a ‘stand for myself’ through his ignorance and authoritarian behaviour.

Through my defiance, he called on his superintendent who came round and contemplated getting a carpenter to break down the door; I continued staying put; by meeting my request I felt, that by using a friendlier manner, I may have ended my protest much sooner.

I felt that with any common sense, he could have started by…

Finding out the purpose of my protest; reciprocating back, I would be detesting the way the foreman was going on about earning bonus. Adding that the way he was coming across was seen as patronising.

By saying my piece, the superintendent could say…

"If he is 'running you down', I will have a word with him. Could you please open the door so that we can talk further?"

Depending on his tone and/or softly, softly approach, I may have answered the door.

In comparison, my protest came with him sinking so low and accomplishing the most devious, despicable and **DIRTY** thing by getting my mother involved.

Back at the flat, the Superintendent replied, "Michael, your mother is here." In disbelief, I recounted, "No she isn't." Sure enough, when she replied, I answered the door and acting stroppy, I could have started 'knocking him about'.

Simultaneously I thought, "How could he have sunk so low and so childish by saying one of the first things when allowing him access to the flat that he could 'smack my bottom'?

With my mother having passed away in 2015, I must strongly make my presence felt by recounting (or saying)…

"Here was my poor mother put through unnecessary stress by this **bastard**; and admitting that he was **that**; this couldn't have been further from the truth and it could have resorted to my mother having a heart attack."

Unexpectedly, he had the audacity to pick my mother up from her home and taking her to where I was working at the time – a flat in Islington.

By writing about events unfolding and being well out of character, nobody else in authority would ever sink so low getting an employee's family involved in a work's protest?

At the time of this incident, autism, it appeared meant nothing to the staff minority; it appeared too, that they could 'walk over' anyone under their authority. The Union however remained weak and was failing to get very far by talking to these 'patronising' individuals, including my 'mate' who I was with almost at the start of my career.

By ending the dispute, the foreman returned with some items of paint, adding that what I did was silly; and talking out loud…

"Maybe so at least my protest I felt, served a purpose and for a short period. Obtaining some 'grace' from his authoritarian tactics."

Afterwards, the supervisor came round, making assumptions that the job was underestimated and, in passing, said that the job needed more hours. By hearing out his assumption that I may have been 'shouldering the blame' through somebody else's error. Adding to his assumptions, I mentioned that a Union appeared non-existent with a stronger recollection that the superintendent was related to it and he agreed.

With things settling down, the peace or break needed from the foreman lasted a few weeks and then, as usual, he reverted back to his usual ways saying that I needed to work faster. This time, and by contracting flu, I felt unable to meet his request and went sick.

LEAVING THE COUNCIL

The beginning of the end on the Council as a Painter and Decorator appeared inevitable. I found it a relief with any 'dented pride' soon forgotten and in its place I was learning new skills at college.

With autism, I failed on the social skills and how to go about my case properly and working my way around my hospital appointments. Already, suffering from back pain following the accident in 1980, I was admitted to hospital with physiotherapy to follow.

When leaving hospital, I found the Council declining to pay for attending the physiotherapy sessions. So I had to extend my sick leave. By having the social skills, I could ask those who I was under, to keep the sessions quiet as one way of working round the issue.

While this was happening, I was under my own doctor with the problem and requested that I should refrain from any bending and lifting. This decision however turned out to be a bad move and, setting myself up for dismissal. I could no longer return to work once the doctor's letter fell into the Council Doctor's hands. I was then put on a probationary period lasting for 12 weeks, hopefully finding a typing position in this time.

As this was coming to an end, the Council were unsuccessful finding the employment that I was hoping for. The only option open, with which I reputedly disagreed, came when the Union Conveyer suggested that I could dispute the Council Doctor's decision. Also adding that I could continue Painting and Decorating once recovering fully from my injuries.

I declined for these reasons…

My pride was already at an 'all time low' with the foreman's behaviour.

Denied promotion by witnessing fellow painters promoted, and 'denting my pride' feeling undermined in the process.

At the tail end of my probation period, a young lad was offered a foreman's position. By 'cringing' at his success, my chances were limited and would have respected the Council by making first contact and finding out whether I remained interested in the position.

In this period alone, my mother had my interests at heart and called the depot on many occasions. She was insisting that I keep my job, with both of us arguing over this issue.

Keeping to my word and saving myself from further loss of pride, I won the argument and started afresh. Eventually, my mother agreed with me, and already she knew that I wasn't happy working for the Council and just as well. Now with some well-deserved freedom, I kept my pride intact along the way.

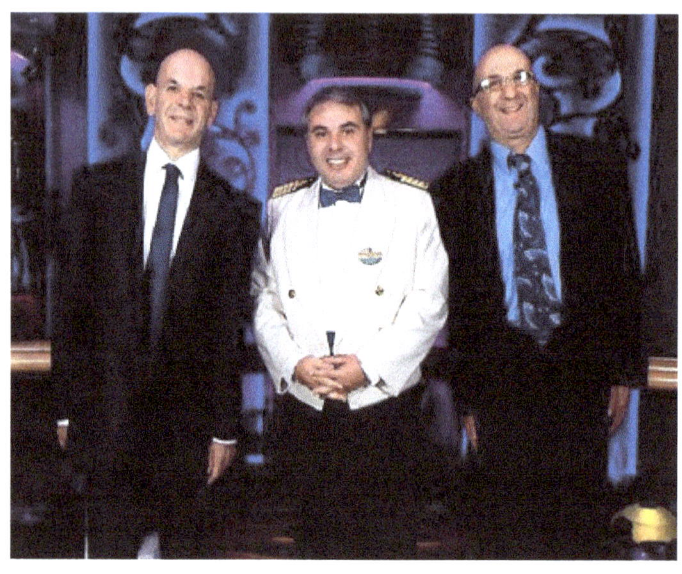

Self with Clifford and the Captain of the ship.

CHAPTER SIX

1. Learning New Skills

On 22nd January I was no longer working for Islington Council. I continued receiving sickness benefit and trying to seek employment in an office-related environment.

When I left the Council, the country was still in recession and in this period one of many Government Training Courses was available for anyone wishing a career change. Ahead of applying, I got to meet the Disablement Resettlement Officer (DRO). His name was Ted.

Under the predicament that I found myself in, Ted was kind and understanding with no time for 'time wasters', or anyone messing around. His goal had to be for his clients to do well trying to obtain employment, gain relevant qualifications and find work.

With the interview getting under way, I mentioned the accident was caused by…

Hurting my back carrying building plant down a flight of stairs and losing my case for compensation as my injuries appeared too minimal in warranting a claim.

Also mentioning my health problems, past employment, qualifications and so on.

Then I went on about working in an office-related

environment while trying to compose myself with a bad cold. I also mentioned that working in an office environment was a privilege. In reciprocating, he thought that this was 'well said' and, praising my willingness to find work.

At the meeting, he touched upon a (TOPS) in Clerk Typing which entailed the candidate passing the pre-entry test in Maths and English before entering the course.

Primarily (or, first) and following Ted's request, he obtained a hospital report surrounding my condition. I could no longer follow my previous occupation as a Painter and Decorator and felt happy giving him the go ahead; with an injured back, I thought it wise performing light duties in admin and continued looking for work in this field.

With so much 'red tape' around at the time, I had to take a short answer test before the Training Opportunities Course. When it came to entering the TOPS pre-entry exams in Maths and English, I failed, and at the same time felt penalised in participating in any of the courses on offer.

Learning the news from Ted, I had two options open to improve my Maths and English – at the local library, or by undertaking a Preparatory Course. I chose the Preparatory Course.

At the start of the course, I felt it useful learning to write various essays and, practising English and Maths ahead of forthcoming exams in both subjects. In between, the atmosphere among teachers and students alike was very relaxed, having a few good laughs along the way and taking part in various outings.

When it came to taking the exams, I felt nervous and only successfully getting the required minimum – 15 marks in English for the Clerk Typing Course; immediately, I started feeling relieved that I passed. As the day progressed, I started feeling much happier by achieving something and gaining valuable knowledge in English in particular.

As the course progressed, the Clerk Typing Course came into conversation I was asked to refrain from undertaking through the pressure involved. So, taking the advice from the tutors, I took the decision by learning to type at evening class and passed Pitmans Elementary and RSA 1 in typing.

Through learning on the Preparatory Course, I felt that the enhanced skills in English and Maths were worth while and reflecting on this…

Seeing my letters published in various magazines; including *Autism London* and *Asperger United.*, an achievement by any means, a teacher on the preparatory course suggested that I write a book; with my grammar at an acceptable standard. I was feeling unsure of her suggestion, as writing a book takes skill and patience.

Returning to reality and ahead of entering the 'real world' in the job market the Preparatory Course included interview practice where I found myself putting myself across atrociously; as I started seeing the video for myself. I returned to the Employment Exchange where Ted, my DRO, gave feedback on mock interviews where I expanded before finding work in an office-related environment.

2. The Job Market

In this section of the chapter, are examples in the discrepancies that I had with various contacts and feeling very resentful at times. So I wished to make my presence felt and, simultaneously, if I didn't have autism and was the placid type, then I may have handled my grievances more professionally.

The Preparatory Course, was the 'crossroads' where the job market existed and learning to type at night school.

Learning this skill I found very challenging, until things made sense as I went along.

In the autumn of 1983, I had already learned to type and secured a position working for Pitfield Youth Centre, North London as a Clerical Assistant filing…

Confidential documents

Allocating external mail to the Centre's departments

Maintaining a member's index file of clubs connected to the Centre

Preparing and banking funds.

This saw a start, gaining experience along the way working in this environment and taking part in one of the many Community Program schemes.

My next position saw me working at a Jewish Community Centre escorting the Senior Citizens home by mini cab and overseeing their well-being in the day.

In between, I had the opportunity at admin work processing Senior Citizens' records and printing and updating Meals on Wheels; sometimes however, I assisted with the Meals on Wheels service whenever the Centre was short-staffed, and helped deliver meals to the house-bound.

As an extra bonus, I saw the chance of integrating with the staff, employees, Senior Citizens and trying to 'better myself' socially. I also enjoyed Wednesday afternoons, their busiest day with more activities on offer, including watching a different entertainer performing each week.

With the skills that I already had, I needed additional office skills and learnt the basics of Word Processing and successfully passing RSA and Pitmans in this skill; over the years, I expanded my knowledge as self-taught in home computing and addressing a certain percentage of PC system issues.

Before getting to the stage of self-teaching or expanding my computer skills, I found jobs in short supply and was signing on at the Employment Exchange until the Employment Training schemes started.

When referred to the now defunct City Training Link (CTL for short) for the training schemes, it was meant to be a start getting back into the job market and saying to myself, "How wrong I was!"

As I went along to the induction, I remained under the impression that they would accept me on my own merits. Unexpectedly, a letter arrived to say that I was no longer wanted. At first, no explanation was given until challenging them where I was told that I was failing by fitting in with the rest of the group.

I was feeling discriminated against with no rights through having an impairment. They disregarded this and, 'adding insult to injury', the successful applicants getting through the scheme were having their photos in the local press.

When a second article appeared showing a group of fresh students successfully attaining their diplomas, I contacted my solicitor for legal advice; my goal was to discredit CTL, asking the local press from refraining publishing further articles, and avoiding a libel conviction.

Today things have changed and, reiterating, discrimination is disallowed against disability and a whole array of other issues, including Age, Race, Sex etc.

Feeling vexed by CTL's behaviour, my problems continued when a small team, our facilitator and I, helped to produce a brochure on…

'1001 ways to handle job interviews' as well as a brief TV coverage and my picture in the local newspaper. The team and I were looking forward to a full-page publication with photos in the local newspaper on completion.

When the project started, the group and I were

distributing our brochures to the local Job Centre and a full-page 'spread' was to be the 'icing on the cake'.

The Facilitator, however, contacted local press without our knowledge and, by chance, I found a small article about the brochure already in the local press. So not knowing how to address the predicament that I was in, I wrote a derogatory reply to the responsible party for failing to keep us informed of her intentions. Eventually knowing that the local press was now unlikely to publish our project in full.

She failed taking things seriously and asked me to call at her workplace. When I arrived, the chances were there for her to act more professionally; offering her sincere apologies and finding out from the local press the chance of a full publication, taking into account any misunderstandings that had taken place.

Her work colleague was adding that I would be sorry by continuing what I was doing. With this attitude, I thought that both were behaving unprofessionally. So, finding out that I wasn't getting very far and with a second reply to follow, I decided on a ploy: Trying alone for publication through a session with the press photographer visiting my home address.

My ploy failed with the paper flatly refusing to publish my picture through that brief article appearing earlier in the year on the subject of '1001 ways to handle job interviews'. So I got to speak to the Editor. Coming over as insensitive, he insinuated that I was 'making a mountain out of a molehill', unaware how he would have felt by anyone stealing publicity from him.

So far, the brochure and City Training Link incidents, are some of many incidents concerning to how I react to certain things.

Following CTL's snub, I had to move to another scheme. This time with NACRO (National Association for the Care and Resettlement of Offenders) and, compared to anywhere else, I was beginning to find almost all Government Training Schemes an 'absolute' farce.

The trainees on the course were learning to type, a skill that I had already learnt, so it felt as if I was covering 'old ground'. No trainer existed and I found the tasks non-ongoing.

With no trainer, the facilitator in charge felt helpless and I took it upon myself to leave through 'hanging around' and doing virtually nothing. NACRO however was free from blame and I must have been having doubts whether the training schemes were properly organised.

For any success coming out of Employment Training, the tasks had to be ongoing. So putting things bluntly, I felt denied with CTL helping improve further the following requisites:

> Interpersonal skills/relationships or
>
> communication between people.
>
> Interview skills
>
> Learning more or improving my admin skills.
>
> A chance learning more or, improving my
>
> social and communication skills.

With NACRO's failure, I moved to a 3rd Training Scheme at Finsbury Park, North London. This time staying for nearly two years.

In between and out of sheer frustration, I was falling out with the Co-ordinator. Similar to NACRO, she too felt helpless by ensuring that everyone was benefiting from the scheme. By acting out of order, or perhaps trying to have a joke at my expense, the time came when she threatened her son to take matters into his own hands. Almost inevitably, this may have happened by upsetting her to the point in making her take any action of this type.

The Co-ordinator seemed unaware of my condition of autism and was continually acting unprofessionally when retorting…

"You're as thick as two planks of wood."

Failing to take her insults, or, the way that she was behaving, I decided on walking off the scheme; on my return, she did apologise. I thought however that her outburst was due to problems that she may have been having outside work, or, lack of understanding my needs, or, my rituals. One ritual I had was working no later than 5pm when a placement became available. The placement I had, meant working until 6.30pm and through this, I was declining the offer.

Making up for my refusal, I went back to college and tried learning a new skill – Audio Typing. A task I found too challenging, and soon I started falling behind in class with the subject too monotonous, typing what was said.

Word Processing however, I fared no better and, 'covering old ground' or, accomplishing tasks that I had already done before. So I left to carry on with the training as before

Towards the end, I decided on setting my own placement at Mind as an Admin Assistant.

This was a break by gaining work experience and performing the following duties…

Typing the Project's correspondence, entering and retrieving their data performance and statistics; writing standard letters; faxing or filing various correspondence items; basic telephone duties.

This placement continued until the end of the Employment Training scheme; so forgetting the 'fallouts' I was having, I parted on good terms with the co-ordinator and staff members.

Between 1991 and 1993, I continued with the placement and signing for work at the same time; I was having periodic work-related interviews at the

Employment Exchange, and getting round to mentioning about a typing business being in the pipeline.

I was again 'at the crossroads' trying to find work and, in 1993, I had my first PC and found that using a Word Processing program was no easy gain as I had hoped. My frustrations trying to master the various tasks were very complicated and only had the basic PC skills to work on.

Out of sheer frustration, I was often phoning the organisation selling the PC and trying to get them to help. As a last result, I contacted the Word Processor's Customer Support Service. In time however, I felt comfortable to the point in trying to start my own typing business. However, I soon found myself unsuccessful through lack of clientele, but an attempt, I thought, was an achievement on my part and securing a friendship with a client along the way.

CHAPTER SEVEN

PROSPECTS EMPLOYMENT AGENCY AND FINAL EMPLOYMENT

1. Personal Development

As a choice to signing for work at the Employment Exchange, I started signing at a newly-opened Job Centre. Soon after, I got to see the Disablement Employment Advisor (DEA). At the appointment, I told him that I had autism and, unable to stay focussed in a working environment.

With the interview progressing, he came up with a former Employment Consulting Agency under the name of Prospects; their aim entailed helping individuals with HFA (High Functioning Autism or Asperger's Syndrome), find work and he put me forward to see them.

When the appointment came, I underwent a Personal Development Program Course at the National Autistic Society which included role play and mock interview practice sessions with two other clients over a four-week period.

One scenario came with a mock argument in a Post Office as a role play example. Learning to accept defeat to the person refusing to go towards the back of the queue through pushing in.

The next stage of the exercise was to undergo one-to-one sessions, interview practice, body language, what to say and inappropriate conversations in the office; so with inappropriate conversations arising, this might involve…

Telling jokes involving 'bad taste'.

Talking about sex.

Politics and Religion, as each of these subjects can incite arguments.

Over-excited talking about 'how many birds or guys' he/she has pulled' over the weekend. And so on.

As a substitution, we were taught to talk about positive things including…

Hobbies and interests

Holidays

Book writing or writing as a hobby

Book writing however is a great topic to talk about and what the book is about; and there are many more sensible topics to talk about. Yet there is much more than putting pen to paper as I was finding out when writing this book.

In the workplace, changes may take place, where a new Line Manager takes charge affecting a Neuro-Diverse contact with autism. This manifests itself with the Neuro Diverse detesting any changes, at the same time being very stressful when the new manager has little knowledge about autism.

When Prospects was around, a support worker was assigned to a certain element of clients, with he or she able to address any issues arising, including change of Management.

On the Personal Development course, a scenario arose in a working environment on shift patterns. This scenario was clearly showing when my reaction was tested in a mock work change predicament and adapting to this environment.

My attitude to this was negative and Anthea, my support worker, and her partner thought that I should be more subtle; so hearing out the alternatives, I may have raised the issue in the possibility for the shift patterns affecting my health, or, coinciding with any important appointments.

With the PDF sessions coming to an end, I joined Prospects where I was given guidance on work, matching my suitability and helping with application forms.

By the time I joined the PDF in 1998, autism was getting to be well known. I had a diagnosis, and Anthea suggested mentioning about my autism in my job applications and at every interview I was attending.

With the correct guidance, I had more success getting interviews. I did very well at some of the interviews and, at one Anthea thought that I put myself across better than the mock interview itself and immediately I perceived this as a compliment.

With time and with perseverance, I obtained a filing clerk post with a building consultants firm. A different DEA saw the position advertised for a disabled person and immediately put my name forward by contacting Prospects.

Gail, another advisor, attended the interview with me and I soon got a call back from her, learning about my success.

2. Last Job

When I started working for the Company, I came into a backlog of files ready for filing and was taught the procedure by getting everything in the correct order.

That first day, I had Anthea, my usual support worker, working alongside by ensuring that everything ran smoothly; before starting, the Line Manager introduced us to her employees and I was given instructions on the methods accomplishing each task.

The job itself consisted of each file having an allocated title and subsections for the various jobs undertaken. Most files consisted of large volumes of paperwork and my job oversaw me ensuring that each subsection stayed in chronological order.

Separate to this I saw myself periodically re-labelling the pigeon holes and filing cabinets. As I was getting to know the job better, the support was slowly reduced to one session per week.

With the one-to-one support reduced, I persevered further and succeeded over a period of time by getting the filing under control. My Line Manager was very pleased with my progress; I was doing so well, that I was limited to how many folders and dividers I could have each week. Little knowing however, that with the job a huge responsibility that various files were going astray.

As part of my autism, I was hardly happy unless both sides were clear at the end of the working week. On a good week I could achieve this result without fail. Each Monday, an additional amount of paperwork existed in the pigeon holes and it took until the end of the week before achieving the same result as before.

In the beginning I found this part of the job frustrating, experiencing unintentional 'fall outs' with an employee. Anthea thought that this was due to a personality clash, resulting in a near sacking through one of my outbursts.

Almost coinciding, I had also lost my sister, Barbara, and more inevitably cumulating in things going wrong. My Line Manager who was of the 'austere' type, heard about the missing documents and asked me to locate them by going through the whole filing system. The filing system was in such a mess and beyond my control. I was unable to locate some of them going astray, resulting in losing my position as a Filing Clerk.

Anthea, my original support worker, must have tried explaining my circumstances and that the files were probably going astray through having lost Barbara and, losing concentration in the process.

By taking my fate well and other than being taken by surprise, I tried finding further employment through Prospects; through permanent rejections, Anthea thought that I should go permanently sick.

The task of trying to find work was a lost cause through poor social and communication skills and numerous health problems; my days trying to find work were over with the doctor writing on the certificate, 'Indefinite Autism'.

CHAPTER EIGHT

GETTING INTO FURTHER TROUBLE

In between my working life, I was getting into further trouble. By sharing the incidents taking place, it means that others can learn from my experiences.

As I was approaching my mid-teens, working in between and trying to understand how Society worked, continued to remain confusing. I was yet to know about the 'real world' and what was expected in the generation that I grew up in. So as part of the learning process, I desired to be accepted by other people.

Making a start, I joined a youth club in Finsbury Park. A club specialising in members with similar problems to mine. I hardly knew what autism was, and I saw myself as ESN (Educationally Sub Normal). Today, this is perceived as a specific learning difference (SPLD).

With little help out there having to fend for myself, I had no choice trying to relate to people or end up an outcast. The club however had members with either an SPLD or maladjusted tendencies. I soon found this out by trying to copy the way a member danced and almost getting a 'pasting' from him. So, thinking that I was taking the p**s,' I had to stop.

In time and getting known better, he 'mellowed out' and perhaps at the same time, trying to find out more about what I was like. By the time I started attending the club, it served a purpose and in the process I was getting to know a female contact, Anna and for a brief period. I had a close relationship with her. She also had special needs and, appearing more immature, I felt unimpressed – including her belching in public. However, the turning point in ending things came when Anna had to stay indoors.

Immediately, I failed using my initiative by staying indoors with her. Before leaving, I was asking her to see me at the next club night. On leaving, I started walking all the way home from King's Cross, saving the return fare money home. The 1½ hours' walk did some good; at the time, I had this thing about my reluctancy paying the return fare through making wasted journeys to places.

At this time and failing to 'stop in' with Anna, it was already dark and her father may have understandably been wary of any undesirables hanging around. Anna, I thought, was fine to a point and felt that I should have Anna with her longer.

As the year progressed, I was successful making new friends locally with a couple of lads who may have had maladjusted tendencies themselves. The run-in I had with them involved one of their female friends.

Unaware of my conduct, I immediately tried kissing her and she started crying in the process. I was however soon to find out that both my friends were failing in taking things lightly, which resulted in them hitting me with sticks.

When left to recover, I refused to back down and I tried getting my own back by threatening them with a large cane from a distance. I noticed one of them carrying a bottle for protection and decided to copy this lad until approaching him where I had to drop the bottle or, face the chance of getting badly hurt.

Finding my pride dented, I had to face the humiliation in front of onlookers witnessing the incident unfolding. Since this incident, I met up with one of the lads again in the late 1970s by having a relationship with his sister, Joanne; mentioning briefly about the incident, he felt fine but taken aback, I believe, he felt unable to comment further about the incident.

The other lad, his old friend who I had the 'run-in' with at the same time, was no pushover. When he was at school, I heard about him rebelling against one of the teachers when getting told off for something.

Resuming the events unfolding in this period, the female contact I upset previously had violent tendencies of her own which I was soon finding out with her lashing out.

Leading up the showdown in the autumn of that year, I was associating with some local lads. We had our own clique and, through our age, we were getting up to much mischief. Nearby, I saw one fellow gang member sneaking up from behind and kissing this female contact while she wasn't looking. At first and 'getting in on the act', I started acting up as a 'bit of fun' ahead of turning nasty.

Back at the house where I lived, she came round with some of her friends; at least five contacts (including herself). Outside the house, all the contacts were lining up in single file and I was asked by one of her friends to 'single out' my favourite ones; I chose this particular contact and another girl.

By trying the same thing, I kissed her as before until she started hitting me and at first I thought that she was joking. As the beating progressed, I realised that she wasn't messing around. However, and recovering from the pasting, I soon started getting my own back in a separate incident.

One night, I had some friends round at my house. One of them suggested that I should 'stand up' to anyone showing disrespect. Some, who I 'hung around' with, thought that I was probably odd and thinking no better than taking the 'rise'.

This same contact who I was giving the 'pasting' a few days previously, was present; she was saying something untoward before I started kicking her in the private parts and in return, throwing bottles. Very soon, I went up to her and knocked her 'spark' out by giving her a hard slap around the head. My actions taught her a lesson, stopping her violent episodes.

With her showing more respect, my sister Josephine was filling me in that she was involved with a separate confrontation with somebody else. Now no longer around, it gives me the opportunity to say that she was no 'pushover'.

Whenever I look back on the event unfolding outside my house, I can generalise a better way of handling things differently; this is how…

Singling out my favourite individual(s) and try talking to them normally and refraining from kissing and, at the same time, preventing any violent confrontations from arising.

With the experience mentioned, I felt as if I was on a learning curve and, in between, I felt lucky to have any girlfriends. Including when I was still at school and by far, I wasn't the only contact. The lucky ones with girlfriends back home were writing expressions such as:

SWALK (Sealed With A Loving Kiss); BOLTOP (Better On Lips Than On Paper); ILY (I Love You) and so on. Calling from a phone box at the weekends, and away from the normal routine while at school.

So far, the two precedents are normal practice and it was safer than trying to 'pick up' contacts off the street. By adopting a sensible attitude of mind, some dance or pub venues being safer.

As soon as leaving school, I was left near enough 'fending for myself' in the 'real world' for much longer and taking longer gaining extra friends. So 'tiding' things over, I had Allen and Leslie living opposite, in between seeing the friends that I already had. I still had my ongoing problems relating to people, or, going the wrong way about things. Including getting into trouble one night when I was in the park with my family, flying my kite as usual.

A short distance away, I saw a group of lads congregating by the shelter. My mistake, and quite commonplace for autistic individuals, is staring and getting into trouble in the process.

One of the gang members had a girlfriend and, looking on, I saw one of them kissing and staring ahead was a recipe for trouble brewing on the horizon; sure enough I soon found out.

A short time period arose ahead of a 'frosty' reception, from a distance. I found the same gang members nearby; in five minutes or so, I was seen. One member approached me, then in an unfriendly manner, asked…

"Do you remember me?"

"Yes," was my reply.

"You tried to take my mate's girl. He's going to punch you in the eye," before making off and rejoining his mates.

At around the same age, I could have seen these lads acting more appropriately or 'brushing aside' any wrongdoing on my part. Another option may have worked by offering the guy an apology to pass on to his mate.

In between, my father diffused the situation, preventing a full-blown confrontation from arising. Sometimes however, trying to walk away from a situation is always wise and sensible.

The nearest I got to anything of this nature was with my sister, Josephine. We had just entered the park and saw these lads coming towards us; using my common sense I walked past, ignoring them at the same time.

At only 16 years of age, it appeared that I was having to refrain from watching couples being close with each other; including seeing the same thing on an outing to Grange Farm Lido in Essex. I almost found myself getting into further trouble looking on at a couple kissing and cuddling.

As a reminder, my father recalled the incident in Springfield Park and prevented an enjoyable day getting spoilt; so I took his advice about looking on and, leaving the couple alone to carry on enjoying themselves on that fine, sunny afternoon.

CHAPTER NINE

ADOLESCENCE AND THE OPPOSITE SEX

1. Starting Out In The Real World

I found integrating with female company very hard compared to the average teenager, resulting with much suffering.

My frustrations were beginning at an early age and 'starting out' in a strange but complicated world. My first encounter about any misfortunes getting a girlfriend came in my early years. The events taking place at Bradstow Girls' School were beginning to fade and now, reality was the real alternative. I had to move on and experience mixing in the 'outside world'.

At Broadstairs, it felt natural joining Polly for a dance and perceiving things as an extra bonus trying to say something worthwhile. Now, and having to adapt to associating with people 'outside' I found was no 'easy gain'; I was about to find out with my first attempt at a ballroom dance venue in the Christmas holidays, finding the clientele the wrong type or too old.

With the ballroom dancing less forthcoming, an opportunity arose by visiting a Boys' and Girls' Jewish Club in East London. I was with a family member when, halfway up the stairs leading to where the club members were associating, I started saying out aloud, "Where are the girls?"

I was oblivious or unaware what the present members were thinking by calling out in this manner, finding this unusual coming from someone visiting the club for the first time and acting unnaturally. The members however seemed friendly enough but, unsurprisingly, I found things very strange and felt isolated. I felt uncomfortable and took it upon myself to leave after 'seeing through' the second visit.

With confidence lacking and feeling so inadequate, I found it too hard making proper conversation in this unfamiliar environment; Josephine however, in the late 1970s met my brother-in-law there in 1976 and made many friends from the club too which opened up their lives.

Now, I am saying to myself, "I wish I could have emulated their success," in comparison to a sad reflection that I was unable to fit into this environment and see my communication skills improve.

Feeling left out, the Christmas holidays were drawing to a close. So Norma, my sister, recommended a venue at Leyton Baths. Norma had heard about the venue previously and so I went with her on that first visit, finding out where the dance was held.

When we arrived, I asked some female contacts to dance, only to find that both were meeting their boyfriends later that night; as things were 'sinking in', I had to start 'getting real' with myself. This was now the local community, and not Bradstow Girls' School where it appeared much easier trying to talk to female contacts.

That first night at Leyton Baths was the beginning of my troubles, and I remember vividly the events unfolding. With the evening progressing, I saw a couple French kissing and both clearly enjoying themselves in the process. The jealousy and emptiness inside was tremendous. Very soon however it was only a matter of time experiencing my frustrations and heartaches to come.

In between and making up for the disappointment on my first visit, the second visit saw some old Southwold contacts attending including a former classmate, Linda. She had the looks and was cheeky too.

Knowing her previously, I found talking to her almost natural; at one point, she had the audacity of asking for a kiss by saying, "Give us a kiss"; feeling speechless and bewildered, I could see that she was joking with her 'coming out' with that comment.

Simultaneously, those who knew me previously, may have seen that I had a disability and, being kind, I soon felt welcomed. With the friends I had back home, I could have gone about asking them to join; through my impairment, I felt my chances were blown or I may have stood a chance getting near enough to my chosen partner.

As the evening wore on, I decided on leaving the dance earlier than usual to find a pleasant evening ending up, spoilt…

With the dance over, I made my way to the cloakroom to find that I had lost or mislaid my ticket!

While trying to explain the loss to the cloakroom assistants, I saw their attitude as off-putting. With few patrons queuing, they had ample time trying to help find my coat. With their attitude, they seemed patronising and lacking the respect that I deserved in the process.

Both were middle-aged and showing ignorance by any standard and I was put to a disadvantage. Choosing by acting reluctantly to search for my coat, I found myself constantly pestering them to act before having my coat returned having given its description by which to go for.

With the relevant social skills, it could have seen me reporting them to the Manager, but I was lacking those relevant skills and appearing that I was 'nothing' through whom I was and perceiving this as so upsetting each time I look back. So 'feeling shy' of a repeated performance, I refrained from attending Leyton Baths until the spring.

So far, my attempts trying to find someone at various

venues remained unsuccessful. So I was introduced to an Iranian girl by a family friend, a contact living with us at the time. I was already very choosy, and going out on a 'blind date' came the 'turning point' as less forthcoming, resulting in trying my luck elsewhere.

The Easter break was starting, and when I entered a nearby local church I saw someone appearing to 'strike lucky' with at least seven girls. Short of trying to evaluate the situation or, failing to observe for long enough, almost immediately I asked one group member…

"Are they his girlfriends?"

He must have been taken aback, knowing how to address my reply as the girls were part of his group; with this odd remark, he too may have thought of me as naive or lacking judgement. So it appeared obvious that the element of patrons attending were the wrong clientele. So, returning to Leyton Baths that same night, with no friends for company may have been unwise with the predicament I had, with an element of thoughtless contacts.

At the venue, I approached four female contacts already on the dance floor when one tried using flattering tactics and remarking…

"You're very good looking," and "You're a very good dancer."

At the back of my mind, I felt the least impressed with this individual trying very unsuccessfully by appeasing or 'beefing up' my self-esteem. With the intelligence I had, I knew that striking up a relationship was virtually non-existent.

Anyone nearby may have told these contacts where to go. On my part, and using the right initiative, I may as well have tried giving them a 'wide berth' by walking away or at least abstaining from leaving the dance with them.

At the time, I felt none the wiser and perhaps, thinking that I was on to something. So, with the quartet and I getting the bus back to Hackney, I found the same girl continuing to poke fun, trying to cause me embarrassment in front of the bus conductor by saying that I was very good looking.

In the process. The conductor may have been thinking one of two things…

> Quipping to her, "You're well in there," with the joke on her.
>
> Finding it strange coming from an unknown contact, not knowing what to say and being taken aback in the process.

With no comment, he carried on his job as normal.

When the bus arrived at Clapton Pond, I left the quartet to make my way home. With the notion I had with those involved, I had no chance with those poking fun at my expense.

Returning to Leyton Baths the following week, my expectations came true seeing two of the quartet members 'paired off' with partners. Adding 'insult to injury', came approaching one girl, asking whether the partner she was talking to was her boyfriend. Her reply in a rather bolshy way was, "Yes, he is, so you better go away."

I thought that her behaviour was so low that she could not get any lower even if she tried. So far, I felt lucky enough to 'rise above' their 'insensitive' actions poking fun at somebody with an impairment.

Through autism, I felt that I had it 'worse' than most teenagers. Hardly able to 'blend' in with a certain element of clientele I also found very upsetting, as much as anyone in my predicament would.

Through being young and sometimes immature for my age, I met with another two of the quartet members again many weeks later. This time she was asking if I could lend her money to repay her teacher. At the time, my mother was doing some shopping nearby, and I very foolishly told her, "There's my mum. I'll ask her if it's fine to lend you the money."

Taking my mother's advice, I didn't part with any money. Seeing this individual for the last time two months later, she carried on with her 'ploy'. All along, I felt that this individual and her friends were still trying to 'have fun' at my expense or with anyone disadvantaged to them. It appeared that with what little intelligence I had, I ended up better for declining from parting with any money.

2. Cousin Sally

Leaving behind my experiences at Leyton Baths, I decided to move on with my frustrations trying to get a female contact as ongoing; perhaps I may have struck lucky with my cousin Sally who I found attractive; so, around the Easter period, my aunt Sarah was holding a Seder Party – an event celebrated by the Jewish religion around the Easter period.

At the party I soon started paying much attention towards Sally. And, with her short hairstyle and attractive looks, many a 'fella' could easily end up 'falling for her'.

At 13, Sally found herself reluctant; 'falling shy' by getting together with anyone taking a fancy towards her. Feeling too young, she needed more time to herself. So, striking a successful relationship appeared a lost cause.

In this same period, she also had a cousin having the same feelings towards her; failing to show any feeling, I felt saved from any discomfort caused and resulting by leaving early.

Things did however turn out in my favour with Sally giving me a friendly smile and was one of my first recollections of flattery. And deviating from the subject briefly…

Another recollection came when 'wolf whistling' to a passing female contact along the street, and she gave me a wonderful smile. She had short brown hair and looked attractive too.

Reminding me of this brief encounter, was a song, 'Don't Bring Me Down' by Eric Burdon and the Animals and has stuck in my mind ever since.

Sally however was visiting my aunt for a second time and I took the opportunity of seeing her once more. To begin with, I started behaving normally until leaving. Then it appeared that I failed by 'picking up on the cues', unaware that Sally may have been shy, by briefly, kissing her on the cheek.

Taken aback, she asked, "What's that for?" I could have added that it is usually seen as 'customary' for families to kiss one another. My aunt Sarah must have thought this as normal. Sally failed seeing it that way and failing also, that I had autism until I made it known to her later in life when she eventually began to know what it meant. Previously, and putting aside that 'innocent kiss,' I acted more strangely towards her in my younger days by…

Stroking her hair in my younger years, to the point that she felt she wanted to cut short visiting my mother. When Sally was much younger and about 9 or 10 years, it was explained that my fascination with girls with brown hair, was one of my passions.

Today, it's looks and, women with smooth or short hair. Over a certain time period, I offered my apologies to Sally.

At 15, my behaviour might have improved as far as my fascination with girls with brown hair goes. Sally now, was seeing things in a 'different light' with my autistic tendencies at my Grandparents' Golden Wedding Anniversary celebration in Mare Street, Hackney.

When the family arrived at the venue, I was placed on the same table as Sally. Suddenly, and unaware of my conduct, I told Sally that she was very good looking, causing her embarrassment; she carried on socialising as normal with my cousins on the same table.

Two cousins, around my age, may have known before of my impairment and brushed aside any embarrassing compliments towards Sally. By now, she too, must have been accepting who I was, before any infatuation I had on her, was about to fade.

On the lighter side of things, she still recalls an incident arising over a bottle of tomato sauce…

Failing to check to see that the lid was firmly tight, I shook the bottle. Suddenly, the lid flew open with the sauce going everywhere with some of the contents landing on Sally. Witnessing this event first-hand, saw everyone laughing.

In time however, the soft spot for Sally started to diminish or fade further until it was no more and now, I was 'at the crossroads' not just with female contacts, yet with trying to relate to people in general.

3. Trying my luck while on holiday

Primarily part of getting on with people is learning to communicate effectively. At the age I was, I wasn't helping my cause by acting inappropriately with perfect strangers. At the time, I was into flying kites and mainly by the sea; sometimes the kite would fall out of the sky and leave a trail of string along the beach. This saw the unfortunate few getting their feet caught in the string.

Failing to compose myself properly, I cursed and shouted at the perpetrators and calling them 'clumsy'. I felt unable to stop and think and pass on any apology. Knowing much better now, I can handle things better in this respect.

At the time, my family and I were already on holiday in Cliftonville and, with a dance taking place adjacent to our guest house, I felt that it was worth giving things a try.

With the dance in full swing, a live act was appearing. So, a family member accompanying me appeared a wise move in the event of anyone trying to be 'funny' and 'picking a fight'.

To begin with, the band was playing at a moderate pace until slowing things down and I asked a girl to dance. Failing to know any better and with my autism clearly showing, I carried on dancing at a steady pace compared to holding her. She must have thought this strange on my part. She too may have had a boyfriend who appeared to observe us. So trying to 'get off' with this individual may have been very unwise under the setup element of clientele.

For the remaining time, we observed what was going on until the pinnacle of the evening came with me besotted with jealousy seeing a selection of males snogging their girlfriends. They were all older than me, yet despite this I found it made no difference.

As we left the dance, I started feeling better. Perhaps however the venue was unsuitable and I may have fared better attending venues with clientele with the same impairment as me. Except, none existed then and, talking about autism, then back in 1966, was pointless with little or no support out there at this particular time.

Still having to fend for myself, two opportunities arose trying to attract female company of, or around, my age.

Unexpectedly, a female contact replied saying, "Hello." Failing to answer, I ignored her. My head was still 'messed up' with the frustrations relating to female company that I was unable to 'bring myself' confidently enough by talking to her.

I was yet to gain the 'know how' to relate to female company and learn the knack of holding down a conversation. Perhaps with a 'sounder mind', I may have had similar luck with the family and their younger daughter…

At the time, my family and I were making our way towards the sea cliffs when my father saw a family with a younger daughter coming towards us. As they got nearer, he said, "He likes your daughter." As usual, I failed to say anything. Perhaps, either through shyness or, lacking in confidence; perhaps if my own family had spoken more to the girl's family, I may have had time composing myself, 'picking up' enough encouragement to 'break the ice' with her.

Coinciding with the contact made, a song, 'Sweet Talking Guy' by the Chiffons, reminds me of the time when this individual and I, could have 'got it together'.

Whatever frustrations I had by being so 'choosy' on the type of female contact that I was after, I wasn't prepared to give up that easily before trying another venue on our second holiday to Great Yarmouth.

This time, and with no guidance, I went along to a nearby venue to try finding out if it attracted a younger element around my age. My plan was to observe nearby, the clientele attending.

At 15 years of age, I saw nothing wrong by sitting in the foyer, but it may have been more wise observing the clientele from a safe distance outside the venue. My decision however observing these individuals attending caught the attention of the Manager looking on at a distance.

Approaching me to where I was sitting, he expressed in an impudent manner, "What are you doing? Are you trying to pull a fast one?" Taken aback, I was unable to assert myself where, finding out whether those attending were near my age, that he may have done one of two things…

> Asked me to leave and failing to 'hear me out'.
>
> Listen to my concerns about whether or not, any clientele around my age were attending and allowing me access.

The Manager however may have had other thoughts, thinking that I was trying to 'sneak' in without paying. Once the Manager said his piece, I decided to leave; but by observing long enough, I found out that the venue attracted patrons older than myself and I had to find elsewhere where the clientele was nearer to my age.

So far, writing about these events is good enough to perceive most of the population's lack of understanding at that time about autism and how it can literally 'blight lives'. To this point, I was struggling trying to find someone until, striking lucky with someone that I continue to remember now. That contact is Moira who I met skating alone at my next venue – an ice skating rink.

Looking as if my luck was about to change, I made contact saying…

"Would you like me to take you round?"

"Yes," she replied.

As we were skating, I started asking loads of questions, like a Police Officer questioning a crime suspect. In the duration, we were getting on fine and soon found the 'inevitable' happening for real…

A date to follow the next day.

At the end of the session while changing into our normal footwear, her younger sister, Hilary, replied, "I bet you love her." Using my common sense to Hilary's comment, I failed answering, or for argument's sake, I could have reciprocated back…

"Yes, your sister is extremely good looking and I love her very much;" choosing by acting sensibly, I kept quiet, averting any embarrassment on Moira's part and saving the friendship so far.

As we were handing our skates back, we soon made our way towards the guest house where we were staying. This time, holding Moira's hand, I introduced Moira, her father and Hilary to my parents.

That night my parents were pleased. By experiencing such euphoria, I was unable to help feeling so 'romantic' and, in passing conversation, my mother 'chipped in' by saying…

"If you behave sensibly enough then you will get a girl." At the 'spur of the moment' however, I was seeing this as a real achievement.

So far, this romance is nothing 'out of the ordinary' for any teenager starting adolescence. Except, and with my autism getting in the way, came a 'twist'…

As Hilary and her father were spending time with my family on the beach adjacent to Yarmouth Pier, Moira and I went to a nearby funfair. So far, things were normal until asking questions that may have been looked on as inappropriate…

Following the time spent at the fair, we walked along the beach and I started asking Moira when she first had a boyfriend and whether she kissed any of them. Her reply was "Yes," and following through, ""Would you like to kiss me?" before kissing her briefly on the lips.

By having my time again with Moira, I could at least have tried letting the conversation flow more naturally, for now and finding a reasonable spot, I had my first real kiss with her and saying to her how much I loved her in the process.

In passing, Moira replied, "Isn't it nice being beside the sea?" But I was failing to reciprocate or 'throwing back' the conversation as in…

"And it's nice being with you."

I felt that at 15 years of age I could at least have tried making an effect using my communication skills more wisely. Something was missing which showed as we were making our way along the end of the promenade to our respective families staying at a nearby beach.

When we arrived back, I told everyone how we kissed, or, to a finer point, 'You know what we were doing?' That was my undoing and my own fault; by keeping quiet, Moira may have shown up later that day or on the last night of our holiday.

Things however may have been more forthcoming by acting neuro-typical; sometimes, having a relationship is far from easy by demonstrating so far my experiences with Moira.

At the end of the holiday, I felt 'lovesick', constantly

thinking of her and lasting long enough for a 'close call' by almost getting into a spot of trouble…

One warm September night, my friends and I were hanging around opposite a block of flats; by the flats was a guy of around my age, or slightly older, snogging his girlfriend.

Wishing that Moira was by my side, I relayed my feelings to my friends. Then, listening in to our conversations, the guy suddenly gave chase until arriving home. Then he left me alone. So giving the reasons for his actions, I cannot perceive what I did was wrong. In narrating my comments the way I felt towards Moira was normal.

Today, I always have time to listen to a Motown classic by the Isley Brothers, 'I Guess I'll Always Love You.' So whatever pleasure I had with Moira, this song always comes to mind and the memories continue to 'shine'.

When the relationship finally ended, I remained free from any emotional upset and, in her letter, she wrote that she felt too young to be having boyfriends and wishing me good luck for the future. So coinciding with Moira's departure, I continued having a much bigger crush on somebody living nearer to home.

CHAPTER TEN

FRUSTRATION OVER A FEMALE CONTACT

1. First Contact

One day, I happened to be doing my family's shopping and passing the grocer's as my first 'port of call' when an attractive girl entered the shop. She was amazing with lovely brown eyes and long brown hair. Immediately, I fell for her and would have loved to have had the front trying to strike up a friendship.

At the time, I was unable to find anyone better and started witnessing history coming before my very eyes and it's still vivid in my mind more than 50 years later.

Like many in my position, thinking how to begin, I was wishing to be the 'forward type'. Whatever I tried saying to her, probably may have been less forthcoming, or coming out with the wrong things. So, with confidence lacking, I finished off doing my mum's shopping and making my way home and constantly thinking of her at the same time. So with the 'Catch 22' situation that I was already in, I literally felt besotted with her and wondering what I should do next?

I was often visiting the shops, and when it was my turn to be served by the shopkeeper, he gently tapped my arm and that may have prevented Anne observing me staring at her.

As part of my autism, she saw me for the first time when I stood outside the shop with my back against the wall and waiting for Anne to come out; as he came out of the shop. As she walked past me, I tried giving her a friendly smile and in the process she abstained from smiling back. Perhaps she thought of me as either eccentric (odd) or a threat and carried on walking past.

Sometimes her younger sister, Jane, accompanied her; my sister, Josephine and I were to nickname her Plaitty through having plaits in her hair.

Unaware of my act of stupidity, Jane may have walked out the shop first and in the process she may have seen me as a 'weirdo' or positively, frightened; seeing the 'bigger picture', I could see Anne getting violent or turning nasty and in return seeing myself self-harming or ending my life by doing something stupid.

So far, I was seeing her as easy-going and short of the violent kind, or, I could have foreseen it affecting my life. Including constantly thinking of this scenario and inevitably sectioned to a lunatic asylum as a real prospect arising.

Mental Health, in addition to autism, was also misunderstood by a cross section of society; today mental health appears more prevalent and I feel that more should be done to prevent for example, some self-harming.

This was the grim reality and I am unable to emphasize enough, the detrimental effect of this scenario having an effect on one's life. And, more than 50 years on, I perceive this period as a vivid and haunting reminder of my early teens.

Focussing back to this period and trying to 'get noticed', for the wrong reasons, I was often saying to my mother…

"What do I say next time I see that girl?"

"Nice day," was to be my reply; an opening line in sunny weather.

Remembering this period, I could easily recall, 'turning the clocks back,' and seeing myself looking at things differently and making first contact as in…

"Hi there. I've been seeing you around quite often. You must be local."

With my nerves 'getting hold', I found it impossible trying to 'build things up' and, out of frustration. Constantly thinking of her and simultaneously unable to get her out of my mind. What could I do?

The opportunity of striking up some conversation was there such as…

Helping with her shopping when she had a full basket and offsetting the load by carrying some of it in a rucksack.

With such frustration, I saw two more 'ice-breaking' opportunities arising – wasted through nerves and limited communication skills. The openings were there with a couple of fine opportunities coming my way…

One fine autumn evening, I saw Anne attending to an allotment outside her flats. As an opening line, I could ask whether gardening was her hobby, following things through as a topic of conversation.

As the crush progressed, she bought herself a dog. A cute black poodle and, looking on, I felt Anne 'looked the part' with her black mac, a wicker basket for her shopping, and her poodle walking along the street beside her.

Thinking back on this alone. I could have said. "That's a nice dog you have there. What's his/her name?" or "How long have you had the dog?" And throwing in a white lie, "I have been thinking of buying a dog like that for some time. "Doesn't he/she look cute?"

With any confidence or 'front' trying these opening lines, it may have prevented a forthcoming episode less upsetting, the day before my 16th birthday. So, it is important sharing my feelings in this troublesome period and for others to learn, or taking into account, the ongoing research studies taking place on autism.

2. Lacking Tender Loving Care

I was about to do more shopping for my family when I saw from a distance, Anne chatting to someone with a teddy boy haircut. And, clearly seeing them engaged in a good conversation, as a normal reaction, I was getting very upset in the process.

Unaware of my presence by both parties, I also saw Anne briefly kissing this guy before parting company; as she parted company, she made her way to the nearby shops, meeting up with some known lads.

Witnessing what I saw and talking out loud…

"All I needed, I felt, was TLC, Tender Loving Care from these lads; I would have appreciated their sympathy or, put at ease and reducing my concerns. It failed crossing my mind even trying to make contact and at least averting the following from happening."

On the way home from doing my mum's shopping, I saw Anne approaching and making her way to some more shops. With my nerves 'clamming up', I soon found that as she was getting nearer, I had the feeling of 'emptiness' and lacking knowledge handling the situation.

With any confidence gained, I may tried inviting her to my 16th birthday party; however, I could see things getting much worse with her accepting. With Anne so attractive, I could see her getting 'paired off' with anyone attending and now saying to myself…

"Were my nerves saving any further heartache to follow?"

Today, and no longer facing the predicament that I was in with Anne, I continue feeling very sad when hearing that song, 'Picture Me Gone' by Dave Berry, bringing back such awful memories.

Reaching home, I felt terrible that my family were unable to get me from deviating my feelings away from Anne, and in its place thinking of the pleasant memories I had with Moira a couple of months or so previously.

The party that I was having that night, was coming at a worse time and cancelling it was almost impossible at short notice. With the party getting into full swing, I found myself fancying a contact named Katy; on the slow dances, I was unconsciously squeezing her and making her uncomfortable in the process.

I wanted comfort with things turning round in my favour but now I found that my party wasn't helping things either. Katy, who I also fancied to some degree, had a boyfriend.

As the evening progressed, Katy sat on her boyfriend's lap and started snogging in the process. It wasn't my day and, feeling jealous for a second time within hours, I felt worthless and choosy too, failing to help my concerns.

By coping with my concerns and feeling more the wiser, I could have walked out and tried killing time by walking around and returning home at around 11.00 pm or later.

Worse still, I could have thrown myself under a train. Nearby was a railway track and through taking this action I may have lost both my arms and legs and been confined to a wheelchair through a suicide attempt of this kind taking place.

Feeling inadequate, I knew that Katy's friend, Shelly, showed an interest in me the year previously; with no feelings to show, I found her very popular and, 'hooked up' with 'her chosen guy'. Despite her success at the time, I had no hard feelings and admired her for putting herself about.

With events unfolding, I felt I deserved better and that's what hurts. This was no ordinary teenage occurrence. On my part, I felt 'set up' for long-term psychological damage later in life and today as the evidence shows.

I rely on antidepressants through feeling depressed, occasionally feeling disorientated, hearing very loud voices at times and on the 'other end of the scale' suicidal thoughts and occasional disorientation and/or being unable to think straight. In the Appendix section of this book, is also more detailed information on my mental well being.

Now in the real world, I was seeing more of Anne and trying hard deflecting my thoughts with no success. At the 'last count', I heard that she was working at a well-known day nursery in Southend. So with any children coming through nursery with an ASC, Anne must have had more understanding towards autism and perhaps, reflecting back on my odd behaviour. As well as this, I have seen her on Facebook in recent years, looking much different with shorter hair and giving such comfort seeing the way she looks now after all these years.

3. Making Contact

Back in 1966/1967 – it must have been obvious how Anne was thinking about the way I was behaving. With little to go by on autism, she may have made some allowances for acting unintentionally 'silly' towards her and with no exception to these two episodes:

One day I tried attracting her attention by ringing my bicycle bell, whereas, a quick 'hello' would be looked on as more appropriate. In between, I could see Anne 'playing things down' or, seeing the weirdest part of my behaviour.

In a separate episode, she saw that I had a bag of the 1960's band, The Monkees; as I was cycling past, she saw the bag and failing to comment she could have asked how the bag was made.

Since failing trying to communicate with her, something had to be done to 'break the ice'. I continued feeling inadequate, and my next stunt seemed far from impressive by asking a kid living down my road to do some 'dirty work'.

So, as Anne was doing her usual Sunday shopping, I told one kid to…

"Go up to that girl and say, 'Girl in the black coat, Michael fancies you.'"

Unaware that I was using him, he cycled up to her and recited my comment; by using my common sense, I decided to keep my distance; I however felt that I wasn't keeping back far enough with Anne catching sight and knowing that I was 'putting him up to it.'

Today, I can now laugh at my own stupidity; Anne however was far from amused by us acting out of the ordinary.

Perhaps a better way in getting round the issue that I was having would have been trying any opening line about Sandie Shaw's win the night before on Eurovision with 'Puppet On A String'. This was around mid-April in 1967.

So with confidence lacking, I was almost finding this an impossibility. With any hope on the horizon, it would be coming from my mother suggesting how to put my feelings across to Anne and how much I admired her.

So, taking her advice, I was putting 'pen to paper' expressing my feelings for her. Also present and giving the confidence that I deserved was an old friend, Philip, and soon I succeeded in striking up the courage and conveyed to Anne, my letter…

Anne at the time, was coming out of the off-licence when I started saying. "Will you take this letter?" Take aback, she felt amazed to the point by asking me to repeat myself. The second time I repeated myself, she took the letter and made her way home.

In the letter, I told her about my admiration for her and whether any chance existed in meeting up, or going out together; where a better way trying to emphasise the way I felt may have been…

Hi there,
I have seen you around and I admire you. I would like to get to know you better but with my anxiety I

am hesitant trying to get to know people that I am unfamiliar with.
Perhaps when we next meet, I will try making an effort to talk.
Kind regards
Michael

By leaving residential school, I felt that it was very hard trying to build things up. This was my first real experience trying to make proper contact with female company, and as expected, failing by following things through regarding the letter.

By 'going beneath the surface', Anne could see for herself the underlying problems I was having; already I felt the 'cracks were showing' trying to talk to Anne properly.

By guessing what Anne must have been thinking. I had to start 'getting my act together' and, with enough courage the second time round, I started talking to her and finding out whether she had read the letter before trying to ask her out.

But already having a boyfriend, she replied, "I'm going out with somebody."

Immediately, I knew how hard it was going to be taking a let-down. Anne was so attractive, I felt she should have had many boyfriends, where she already had somebody living on the same estate where she lived.

Over a certain period, I was getting to know Anne's boyfriend by selling Useless Eustace tickets to his mother in the late 1960s. In passing conversation, I was learning that when both were very young they often played in the children's play area. When it was time for the boy to come indoors, she often had to call down.

In recalling the concise history between Anne and her fiancé, I am still thinking this as the biggest curse I have heard; with Anne growing up with this lad, nobody so it appeared, stood any chance 'striking it lucky' with her. I was reluctant giving up that easily; by meeting Anne at the local shops and in the presence of the shop assistant, I immediately came out with…

"Would you like to see a couple of horror films?"

Anne, as before, coolly replied, "I'm going out with somebody."

As part of the learning process, I found myself unaware by making a 'hash' of things; now the wiser, that it may have been unwise talking about films; so, part of the process learning 'social skills' I could begin with…

"Hello. Have you had a good week?" or, "How's school?" etc. (And so on.)

With Anne already in a relationship I may have started…

Getting to know her better to the point of embracing her or, giving her a kiss on the cheek; in most social situations, this is achievable and also, as a consolation for one's trouble talking to any fancied male or female.

By writing about these events surrounding Anne, it may be true that some consider this as part of the 'adolescence' or 'growing up' process. Through autism, I felt that trying to act the same as anyone else was appearing was virtually impossible.

I was unsuccessful getting very far with Anne and was thinking of her constantly. She felt so special, but still I had some learning to do. Now, 'word was getting out' about the crush or infatuation that I had for her…

One night, I happened to be walking home from a youth club in Finsbury Park. Suddenly, Anne's older sister, or one of her friends called out from the flats where Anne lived saying…

"You like Anne." Taken aback by this unexpected encounter and not knowing how to address the situation, I reciprocated back, "Who's Anne?" as an alternative to saying, "Yes I do like Anne, is she your sister?"

I seemed lost for words and unable to pursue any conversation. By responding properly, my confidence may have been boosted by seeing Anne the next day. This time, Anne her younger sister, Joy and her friend, Betty were by the flats' entrance.

Passing by, Betty called out and I went towards her and tried striking up some conversation; unable to address things, I replied, "What, what do you want?" Before walking away and not knowing what to say and appearing unsociable. Except, it appeared that I was 'losing the plot' of things; whatever I was doing trying to 'get round' Anne, was consistently, a lost cause or better still…

'Fighting a losing battle' with Anne, with Jane and Betty appearing to be playing things down.

Now in the 'real world' by spending much time at boarding school and perhaps with the right 'frame of mind', things may have been wiser 'hanging tight' a little longer and trying to interact with people better by learning new social skills.

With a lull arising between Anne and I, things started to quieten down until one fine July day; and a glorious day too.

As I was cycling along the road I came across Anne on the opposite side of the road. Suddenly, I shouted out. "Hello Anne!" She reciprocated by giving such a wonderful smile and, emphasizing the point…

"Boy, didn't I feel flattered!"

By walking instead of cycling, I may have ended up giving her a big hug for her friendliness.

By coincidence, The Beatles were in the process of releasing, 'All You Need Is Love'; and, it seemed that with Anne's friendliness, it appeared that I was getting some 'love' again since meeting Moira. I was feeling so elated compared with the way I was for a very long time and longing for this period of happiness to last. I found it short-lived.

4. Further Frustrations

Less than a week with Anne coming over very friendly, I was taking a stroll through Springfield Park one night. From a distance, I was observing a female contact more attractive in comparison to Anne. She looked so friendly and appeared to have a boyfriend receiving much attention from her. As she brushed her hair back, she looked absolutely beautiful.

Seeing this at first hand, I found was very upsetting to the point that I could see the most placid teenager becoming jealous. It seemed very unfair witnessing this by myself. Unable to handle the situation, I came home in a terrible state, feeling empty and feeling like a total outcast. It felt as if I never had anyone but my family for support. I would have loved to have had the social skills trying to approach these people and trying to get some rapport going.

Witnessing this event unfolding, I may have been one of many teenagers in this difficult situation. Anne however and so far, was 'brushing aside' my obsession or, feeling inclined and in a bolshy way, she could have reciprocated saying…

"Go away and leave me alone!"

With a scenario of this kind arising, it could result in being in a limbo position and forced to move on. So with the passage of time and on the proviso that I could handle a scenario of this nature taking place, a severe rejection of this kind may fade over time. However, in truth, I continue having bad memories of Anne and feel it improper pretending otherwise.

At the height of summer in 1967, I was beginning to feel so worthless that I may have been better off staying out of the park before the 'twilight' hours were beginning. Today things are different compared with the 1960s where seeing young couples walking in the park was very common, including witnessing a ginger-haired contact looking ecstatic and witnessing her feeling so happy and being unable to resist constantly hugging her boyfriend.

In passing, I could have recounted (told) this female contact how lucky she was and wishing that I was in the same situation.

At the same time as witnessing these incidents, another brief lull arose with Anne. Through my nerves, following these events…

I was staying with relatives over in South London. On my return, I found myself in a better frame of mind. The weather was favourable too for Anne and her family (including Jane) for attending a concert party taking place in Springfield Park.

Seeing Anne this time round, by experiencing my unfortunate encounters, I found the crush on her previously was less intense. And a good thing too, through seeing somebody better, as the reason.

With any dilemma that I may have been faced with, it appeared that I could either give up any attempts trying for Anne or to continue trying. I opted by trying further with a crafty plan lined up, involving my sister Josephine, following Anne's family attending a recent concert party.

At the next concert party, my plan was trying to get Josephine to make friends with Anne's sister, Jane. Josephine, my sister, must have been around Jane's age and I was hoping for a friendship between them. The stage was set for the stunt where, sure enough we were to strike lucky through the presence of Jane's family.

Jane, by this time had been separated from her family and appeared by a water fountain. Taking the opportunity, I introduced her by saying, "This is my sister, Josephine," and started messing around.

As she stepped up on the fountain, I pushed down too hard on the knob resulting with the water missing her face. I cannot forget the innocent smile on Jane's face, and also it was a perfect moment trying to get Josephine to strike up a friendship.

To my disappointment, the stunt failed. Jane appeared shy and failed to reciprocate back.

At this precise moment, things may have turned in my favour with the stunt failing to materialise and now, more the wiser, I could see things ending as a complete farce; and coming to mind…

Seeing Jane's parents coming to the house instead of Anne before taking her home.

I could also see Keith, Anne's regular boyfriend, collecting Jane from where I was living in the 1960s at Moore Close.

By putting myself in this scenario, I continue shuddering at the consequences. Today, this must be an extremely rare occasion for anyone trying to get their family involved in the frustrations that I was having with Anne so far. So and talking out loud…

"I strongly advise anyone against copying the idea I had in mind, averting any disappointment and/or heartache along the way."

Unobliterated about these scenarios, I anticipated trying the same thing as before when my father intervened and stopped Josephine from going to the park; out of sheer frustration, I started getting very stroppy shouting…

"If they are over the park, I'm going to smash the place up!"

To his displeasure, he retorted. "I'll break you!"

I shouted back. "You shut your f*****g mouth!"

By having the correct social skills, I could at least tried turning around in my favour by saying to my father…

"Dad, I am constantly thinking of Anne and it is stressing me out. If Josephine cannot come to the park with me, then could you please advise how I can turn things round in my favour when she is attending the show with her family?"

Feeling ashamed about the way I acted, I would have loved to have had the relevant skills when I was growing up and at least, trying to alleviate the frustrations that I was having.

As I tried 'cooling off' from my outburst, I attended the show alone and, with luck on my side, Anne and her family were absent; my intentions were however if they were present, was to return home and smash the place up through a wasted opportunity arising.

Very soon the outburst that I was having with my father was forgotten, besides any animosity from Anne's family. Moving on, society has changed and anyone in my position at the time may have got away with the contact's family or boyfriend saying a few 'choice words'. Things however may be different to any 15 or 16-year-old starting out and going the wrong way about approaching women, with a family member or boyfriend being so downright nasty to the individual at fault.

In the 1960s, it felt so far that I was 'getting away' with my untoward behaviour; Anne, who, in character, was always polite. With any respect and admiration I had for her, she was very good at 'playing down' my unintentional antics or any wrongdoing played on my part with one exception…

I was going off Anne more, and seeing that my behaviour was getting a little untoward, decided to 'get one over' at a local bus stop. Hoping that Anne would board the same bus, I tried keeping my distance before finding the ploy failing. I was already seen, and very craftily she got the bus behind the one that I was already on.

I felt slow however picking up on her craftiness but found myself fortunate enough avoiding feeling too upset through liking somebody else – Violet, who looked after Josephine and Barbara, my sisters, in their younger days.

By the time I started acting more appropriately towards Anne, I knew that trying to have any relationship was virtually nil. In the same period, her mother appeared unhappy with the way I was going about things by her showing such contempt, I saw her staring and giving dirty looks from another bus stop.

I felt past caring and a 'blessing' that the crush on Anne was fading through liking this new contact, Violet. At the same time, I started 'broadening my horizons' by attending various clubs and having fun with my friends; including socialising in our locality or going further afield on our bikes.

At last, I thought that I could, for a very long time forget about feeling uncomfortable, thinking of Anne the day she walked into that grocer's shop one sunny August day in 1966.

CHAPTER ELEVEN

A CUT-OUT PICTURE

This period looks back on events taking place in 1971 and through very little judgement that I may have been classed as a little eccentric, even odd. One day, a club leader re-opened a Youth Club in Hackney after a lapse of 14 months. Getting there was only about a 15 minute bus ride.

In comparison to myself, it may have been good for former Club Members having their club back. Where I stood, I found it a big mistake before resuming a 'soft spot' on a girl who was often 'cold' or unfriendly. She had the looks, and I saw for myself the opportunity she and her friend were having by associating with two male club members.

Outside the club, a singer (Clodagh Rogers) came up in conversation. She was about to appear in the Eurovision Song Contest with 'Jack in the Box'. By mentioning her name, the girl asked, "Who's she?" Failing to make any comment as in 'she may have a good chance in winning the contest', I declined answering, not knowing what to say ahead of these lads walking their partners home.

Already feeling uncomfortable, one of the lads sarcastically said, "Bye byeeeee", holding his composure at the same time.

As they were about to leave, I could have taken

exception and started an altercation; I found myself very resentful when attending the club again; I intended hurting this boy through him getting 'too close' to this girl' or, to a finer point, 'snogging' her.

Away from the club, I saw a picture of Clodagh Rogers in the *Evening Standard.* I cut it out and saved it and found myself unconsciously thinking that this girl would 'brush aside' any stupidity on my part.

When she, returned to the club, my words were…

"You wanted to know who Clodagh Rogers was," and very foolishly, showed her the cut-out picture. Her immediate reaction was…

"That's fantastic! he cuts out a picture and shows it to me."

Walking away, I clearly saw her laughing in front of everybody and trying to show me up in the process. In between, I was still feeling undermined by one of the lads showing off; on the same night, I reversed my decision by refraining from hurting one of the lads and 'bottling out'. I decided on the sensible option, leaving the club early to make my way home.

Feeling the worse for wear, emotionally, I was about to send a letter to this club contact about how I felt and what I intended doing to her. With the letter ready to go out, I had a telephone number and took it upon myself by 'having it out' with her parents the next day.

When I got round to calling, her mother answered the phone. Immediately, I shouted. "Is .... in!?" She replied that she wasn't at home. So following things through, I shouted down the phone using a threatening manner, and retorting…

"Tell … [name withheld] that if ever she shows me up at the club again, I will land her one!"

"What?!" her mother replied before repeating myself. Retorting back, she interjected, "If you ever lay a finger on her, you will get two on you!"

Listening to the commotion taking place, was her

father threatening to 'knock the living daylights' out of me. I retorted. "You try!" before being invited round to talk further about her wrongdoing.

Ending the conversation, I wasn't exactly unaware what I would be 'letting myself in for by visiting her parents and inevitably, would be given a 'cold reception', or even a beating from her father.

With enough common sense, I abstained from visiting them and did some shopping and calmed down in the process. Over several days, I saw myself calming down sufficiently enough by writing to the girl's parents and promising that I would refrain from 'having it out' with them by any further incidents arising with this contact.

At the time of writing the letter, I found myself regretting what I did, finding it virtually impossible trying to get something together with the 'contact at fault'. Since this incident however, she continued remaining 'cold' when I came across her working in a pharmacy and giving me a dirty look along the street when catching up with her again in the early 1980s.

My local friends however thought I did the right thing, 'letting it out' on her parents. So, with undivided opinions, I abstained cautiously from returning to the club through the risks of any reprisals from her male friends.

Things in this difficult period were bad enough at work and within my social surroundings and getting much tougher, seeing myself being very subdued with a contact much younger than myself.

CHAPTER TWELVE

FIRST TRUE FEELINGS

By the time I was getting to my early 20s, I was having sensitive feelings towards some, less fortunate compared with myself, or, going through a rough period and reflecting more in the younger generation. Suffice to say however, that I was still acting immature in certain areas as I was yet to mature more.

When I lived in Hackney, I encountered my saddest moment of all surrounding Francis. At this time I was still very young, and in time I got to know about Francis's sad loss of her father; her loss soon had an impact by me 'feeling her pain'.

I first came across Francis the moment she walked into Springfield Park as a nearby show was taking place. She was no more than eight years of age and, before losing her father, I saw her looking subdued then, and, appearing sensitive.

Between June 1969 and September 1971, and because of my own problems, I paid little or no attention in how she was coping throughout this period.

Her popularity however appeared to grow over a game of rounders taking place outside the flats, on fine summer evenings. As a shortcut to my local pub, I often walked through the flats, observing the game of rounders taking place. So, oblivious that there was anything wrong, I carried on with my life as if nothing had happened, until getting to know Francis better.

One day, Francis came over to the house with an older friend, to see some photographs. I was soon picking up on her looking withdrawn through losing her father in 1970, having first previously heard about her loss through my sister Josephine and, finally, through one of Francis's friends ahead of a delayed reaction through Francis's subduedness.

That night, I literally 'fell to pieces' by crying my eyes out for her, unable to believe how I was crying so much. By contemplating ending my life through the pain that I was going through, it may have been wise waking my parents and mentioning any suicidal attempts that I may have had in mind.

With another plan in mind, I waited until the next day and mentioned to my mother how I was feeling. This time, showing compassion towards my ordeal and in comparison, the issues that I was having at work.

By getting to know Francis better and getting over her pain, I visited her mother, Helen and in passing she mentioned briefly about the loss of her husband. So, failing to elaborate, I mentioned how upset I was hearing about her loss. I had the opportunity by telling Helen, Francis and her younger brother, Brian, the pain I felt for poor Francis that night.

With any bereavement, and in the predicament that I was in, I was finding it hard knowing exactly the right words to say after one's passing.

Francis however, I couldn't help feeling sensitive towards her and continue finding this memory very painful, also witnessing two other child-related incidents in this period alone.

A child was hit by a car as I was cycling behind along the road, immediately noticing her unfortunate encounter. With any luck, she must have got away with a few bruises. My immediate reaction was distress, and I stopped to see what I could do to help, with anyone with common sense doing the same.

Fortunately and worse for wear, she was able to get up and, over time, recover from the shock.

Another instance came with another child near enough brain damaged. I noticed her in the chemist's and witnessed her shaking and looking extremely subdued to the point of upsetting the most placid in 'all walks of life'.

I felt that in this short period. I cannot recall being so 'shaken up', with the exception of another upset to come in the next Chapter. Francis fortunately, did get over the loss of her father, and the last I heard came with Helen, her mother, recounting that she was living in Portishead. More recently I succeeded in finding her brother, Bernard on Facebook.

Through forgetting who I was, nothing materialised; one day, I may catch up with Francis to tell her how I felt about the loss of her father, and in comparison telling her about losing my parents and my younger sister, Barbara.

CHAPTER THIRTEEN

DANCE HALL CRUSH

With most youngsters experiencing 'hang-ups' with partners, I appeared to be acting incompatibly. At 21, I still had countless rejections or, was mixing with the 'wrong' type of people. I could go on.

This difficult period has been one of many traumatic episodes that I have encountered and I feel that I must comment on my feelings about this individual.

The contact, Alice, I thought was a very warm sincere person. In speaking terms, "How wrong I was." This is my story and how Alice certainly contributed to my ongoing mental health issues. At the time, I felt very strongly for Alice.

When the 1970s started, I was in my late teens and still having sensitive feelings. The year was now 1972 and was 'rather' turbulent. First, came a crush on a female contact as her family was about to move to Ireland. I was to miss her very much and, to coincide, I was finding that hanging around my neighbourhood was no longer fun on weekends.

As a substitution, I decided to visit The Royal where in the early 1960s, the Dave Clark Five were performing at the height of their fame. I was a huge fan of theirs and before meeting with Alice, I had previously only attended the Royal on the odd occasion or so.

Unbeknown as to what I was letting myself in for, it wasn't long before I came across her and, looking so friendly, I instantly fell for her. She displayed such a warm personality and was looking very trendy with a black woollen jumper displaying a very colourful design on the front.

When we did get to dance, and unaware of the correct manner of going about things, I tried flattering her by telling her how good-looking she was and how the 'boys must be running after her'. She smiled with the compliment given, and this was in between a tune, 'Hold Your Head Up' by Argent.

When the song finished, I should have continued talking. At 21, I was young and today, I can find it very hard trying to hold down a conversation with unfamiliar people. So, leaving her, I walked around the dance hall, listening to the music playing at the time.

Before leaving the Royal, I approached Alice for a second time. This time asking whether I could take her home. This may have been a bad move with her declining. So taking a telephone number may have been the better option or asking when I could see her again.

That night on leaving the Royal, I was unaware of the heartache to follow.

In the coming weeks, I continued attending the club and found her absent each time. I was however lucky to learn that she was from Kentish Town (North London).

With things building up, I was so upset, that I cycled to Kentish Town one warm May evening with no chance of seeing her. I can remember this period well, being alone as well in the house with my family away on holiday.

Things however were no better at the Royal and I had that jealous feeling, seeing a contact snogging someone extremely attractive. Also helping bringing back such unpleasant memories, was a song around at the time…

'Walking In The Rain With The One I Love' by Love Unlimited.

Today, I feel uncomfortable listening to the song and bringing back the bad memories in this given period.

Through being at Kentish Town more often than normal, trying to come across this contact, I knew of a succession of weekly Country Dancing sessions taking place at nearby Parliament Hill Fields. I went along, and at one session I saw Alice watching the dancing with her father and immediately, was thunderstruck. I felt deterred from talking to her through the fear of her father objecting and adding to my frustrations.

Following the session, both of them took a bus and I decided following on my pushbike and cycling the short distance to a nearby location (off Kentish Town Road).

The purpose of this exercise was to see where they lived; so cycling past, may have been very wise in case of being seen following behind. With so much discomfort, I was already overwhelmed with my emotions and longing for this 'pain' and heartache to end.

By finding out whether any solace, or comfort was on the horizon, I thought that a contact would offer temporary relief from the trauma experienced.

One night cycling through Kentish Town, I spotted someone who I thought was the contact that I had a crush for. I spoke to her and, by coincidence, she had the same Christian name.

This solace however wasn't to last long when I was 'lounging around' in nearby Parliament Fields, a few weeks later. I soon realised that I was talking to the wrong person; by coming to my senses, I was visiting this location until the County Dancing sessions ended.

In the autumn of that year, things were to quieten more and in late October, I had a crush on somebody else. One night in early March, 1973 on a visit, I was anticipating her visiting the Royal after mentioning her present attendance.

Returning to the Royal, there was no sign of Alice I saw a few nights previously. Choosing the wrong night,

I was to come across the contact who I had a crush on the year previously and, as before, I found myself equally as besotted with her and approached her. However, as I was about to try talking to her, she literally walked away. Feeling extremely shocked, I saw the night through and came out of the club, feeling very despondent.

At work the next day, came my first suicide attempt with an overdose of Anadin tablets but finding this having very little effect.

At the time, I was a painter and decorator working near an unspecified number of high-rise flats; by feeling inclined, I could have tried entering the roof and doing my utmost by 'striking up' enough courage by 'throwing myself off'. I am now wishing that I could have taken that decision; since the early 1970s, I continue having haunting memories of this period resulting in avoiding Kentish Town at all costs.

Following my attempt, I worked the rest of the day; by the time I arrived home, I told my family what I had done and they were shocked by my decision to end my life. I went to see the family doctor with my mother; when seeing the state I was in and clearly subdued, I was signed off work and, on the doctor's certificate, it showed, 'Anxiety State' and told to drink plenty of water to prevent any damage to my liver.

Since the shock and emptiness inside, my mother booked to see a therapist named Mary Arkwright. This appointment however, I knew very little about; simultaneously, whatever was mentioned, did nothing appeasing my mind. In that week, I had thoughts about trying another attempt on my life. So far, it appeared that there was nothing left in life and that the events leading up to things, the previous year, was a contributor. Including constantly thinking and missing a female contact when her family moved to Ireland.

With the therapy with Mary of little use, my family booked an appointment with a psychiatrist at St

Clement's Hospital, Bow, London. At the consultation, the psychiatrist (and in an audacious way) recounted that I had no right to consider ending my life. I turned round saying that committing suicide was never at any time, illegal. I was thinking that he had no idea how I felt and must have thought that any failed suicide attempt may have seen me Sectioned or sent to Broadmoor.

With this episode taking place, I continued trying my luck and failing to give this contact up completely. I continued attending the Royal and, on one occasion, asking Robbie Vincent, a Radio London DJ to play 'Could It Be I'm Falling In Love?' by the Detroit Spinners as a song associated with this so-called contact, Alice. My ploy however failed and I had no further luck coming across her at the Royal or, at Country Dancing.

In time, my thoughts were soon forgotten until the autumn of 1980 at the Electric Ballroom, Camden Town. Adding 'insult to injury' however, she had a partner with her. Amazingly, I continued fancying her, simultaneously feeling dejected and prevented from making contact with her.

Today, the 'scars' from this period, are still there and I can see nothing changing in the future.

In conclusion. I make NO apologies for exposing Alice for the hurt and pain that she has given me. If she has experienced any heartache herself, then she would have known exactly how I felt and today, I continue to do so as of now. So, I hope that by getting this message across, that lessons can be learnt by the younger generation not to upset anyone to the point, and, risking the individual of self-harming or 'ending it all' as a last resort.

CHAPTER FOURTEEN

DEBORAH

For any neurotypical person, a fairytale episode might not be of relevant importance; with Deborah around and soon falling for her, my thoughts of the events happening at the Royal the previous year were gradually pushed to the back of my mind.

A new chapter was beginning by knowing Deborah well over a four-year period, and over a game of cricket. In recollection, it seemed a privilege meeting with her and alleviating the painful memories in the previous chapter.

Since that hurtful snub back in March 1973, I am taking the opportunity of mentioning Deborah from the beginning and the impact that she had on my life.

This is my story:

Having left my friends after a game of cricket in Springfield Park, I got as far as the duck pond and intended to make my way home. Deborah and her friends were already in the park, and Betty, another friend, asked whether I could lend her the cricket gear following a game with my own friends in a nearby field.

With the game in play, I refrained from making my way home and decided to sit down somewhere. Betty, who I have known since the late 60s, asked if I wanted to join in. My reply was, "No thanks."

Unknowingly, on my part I must have been avoiding any flack through the risk of passers-by making hurtful comments. Including…

"F*****g idiot. Why don't you grow up and stop playing with the kids?"

So I can envisage the embarrassment caused with this scenario existing and that any 'back-chat' to these individuals, may have seen further trouble. Including, the risk of getting hurt.

Since the game of cricket, I thought no more of Deborah until one fine September evening where I saw her coming towards me while cycling past Clapton Common; when she appeared, I was extremely shocked and instantly fell for her through her stunning looks.

Immediately, I could have started by trying to talk to her but then finding her running away through any uneasiness on her part; believing that I had lack of know-how trying to put Deborah at ease was to be a long, drawn-out process and with common sense, I cycled past, waiting for an opportunity to arise before approaching her for real.

At this precise moment however, and compared to today, I am unable to recall falling for anyone else this way ever since. At this time, I was trying to refrain from making any contact whatever. So, deflecting the situation that I was in, I could only say a brief 'hello' as I was cycling past one night, with no response from her whatever.

With no response, things were obvious that I had to be patient a little longer; and, making contact over a favourable opportunity arising in May, 1974.

As Deborah was passing through, I was showing photographs to a group of people; walking past, I asked her if she had a sister in any of the photographs.

Showing her nerves or saying very little, it looked as if 'building things up' gradually was the norm. In the autumn of the previous year, I was getting over the shock of falling for her. Now a long lull was to follow. So by 'breaking things down', I continued associating with my local friends and coinciding, the local youths were getting up to no good hanging around the flats; damaging local property and causing provocation on my part and resulting in retaliating back.

Most of the youths were from their early to late teens. So, by Deborah overcoming her shyness, I could see her 'getting it together' with anyone 'taking a shine' towards her. Including the time seeing her over the common and falling for her, the first time.

In between, I had my own friends and was still working at painting and decorating; most of all, I had a very good family to go back to. Mum and Dad were very understanding and would do anything when met with any difficult periods.

As I carried on my life as normal, I started falling for Deborah for a second time in 1975, by seeing her walking along the street with a friend. She looked innocent enough, showing off her fringe and long brown hair and looking as good since first falling for her 19 months previously. Already I felt that the crush that I was having, was taking my mind off past events taking place in 1972/73.

By the time I started falling for Deborah, for a second time, the local youths had moved on and another new chapter was beginning by making friends with some of them and mentioning one contact…

Terry was one; his crowd hung out at the Swan public house nearby and wasn't trouble to anyone unless anyone tried 'crossing' or going against him; since getting to know him properly, he has always looked on me as, 'being his friend.'

With the crush on Deborah well underway, I found that we were both nervous of each other. I had to find a way trying getting her to feel at ease.

One day, I saw Deborah coming out of a pub off-licence; I was about to enter the pub next door when I replied, "Alright Deborah?"

Taken aback, she failed answering before making her way home, so I was unable to follow things through. This time however and in comparison to Anne, I was no longer ringing my bicycle bell; getting somebody else to tell Deborah I fancied her; displaying a bag of the Monkees; and no more waiting outside the grocer's with my back against the wall.

So, treating things more consciously, I felt determined in refraining from messing up with her in comparison to Anne. In the coming months before seeing Deborah at her house, I was still trying to make contact, with a couple of opportunities arising.

The next opportunity came when I was riding along on my bicycle, and getting near enough for her to hear, I again asked, "Alright Deborah?" and was given a surprised look. I felt shocked and upset. So, a friendly wave may have been more appropriate.

In between this period, a second opportunity came following a game of tennis with friends.

At the top of Springfield, a road parallel to the park, Deborah passed by where I coolly said, "I've been playing tennis with my friends." Feeling 'tongue-tied', I went quiet and she started running off before saying, "See you" where she reciprocated back with the same.

With the predicament that I was finding myself in, it felt that I was taken off guard or, finding it hard trying to keep the conversation going. This was the hardest part, or I could have started off with…

"Hello Deborah, have you had a good day today?"

"I have been playing tennis with my friends; how about you; are you any good at tennis?" Or better still, "Remember that game of cricket with Betty and her friends? Well I bet you prefer tennis in comparison to cricket."

By exhausting the 'tennis subject', one may try elongating the subjects by finding out if she belonged to any clubs; her favourite pop act; any employment ambitions and so on.

Another concept (idea) is the friendly-tone approach and putting her more at ease in the process.

So, unlucky with Deborah passing by, I had a couple of reasons to visit Deborah's mother; visiting her a second time, I was invited in and saw Deborah looking more relaxed. Also, present were her brother, Arthur and her sister, Karen.

Through my nerves, I felt too afraid getting too close to Deborah by holding both her hands, looking her in the eye and adding how attractive she was; and, trying to kiss her too. By trying this tactic, I could see Deborah locking herself in her bedroom and asked to leave by her mother with a possibility of ending any association with her. Through nerves, it felt as if I was being spared of any scenario, arising and 'saving the day'.

By us getting it together however and inviting her round to where I was living, I could see a scenario for real happening by…

Kissing her and rubbing my hand along her leg; some youngsters may have 'tried this on' with their girlfriends and seen themselves withdrawn or subdued in the process by an immediate relationship breakup to follow.

Taking account for myself in this scenario happening for real any further suicide attempt in comparison to my first attempt in March 1973, may have been successful.

So far, things appeared to be looking up. One mild February night in 1976 when associating with a friend, John, living nearby I saw Deborah's family in the distance. As they got near, I said, "Hello." Reciprocating back, Deborah gave such a wonderful smile that I could have gone over and given her a big hug. By accomplishing this, it may have prevented an instance in clamming up when trying to talk to her again in the company of her friends.

By this time I was getting known better by Deborah and clearly saw my nerves showing when trying to talk to her in the presence of her friends. At the age that she was, I could have perceived her getting together with any male contact to her liking; this did not happen until later while, shyness on her part, appeared to be holding her back. Despite this I did have my suspicions that she may have had a boyfriend and as a normal reaction, seeing myself in complete shock and to the extreme, taking exception by getting into a fight. More than likely coming off badly hurt in the process. I was never really the aggressive type and perhaps would not have had any confidence taking any action of this kind.

With the summer arriving, we saw one of the hottest ones on record. So apart from knowing Deborah over three years previously, I also got to know two of Deborah's friends, Joanne and Rosie by visiting with a friend, Mick.

Already I was having doubts about Mick trying to forge a friendship with Deborah and asked him to refrain from doing so, with Deborah having her hair cut shorter and looking less attractive. This, however, was a wise move on my part ahead of another lull arising.

When she started growing her hair back, I found her looking as attractive as before; so, with Christmas almost getting near, I thought about asking her whether she would be willing to accept my invitation to a family Christmas party.

Ahead of the party, a cousin of mine was due to attend and my suspicions were aroused with him forming a friendship with her. My thoughts on this premonition along with any suicidal thoughts I had, caused much friction with my family until Deborah started turning down my invitation.

With further friction prevented, it may have been 'a blessing in disguise' and saving the atmosphere from 'turning sour' with things appearing to turn round in my favour.

In early 1977, with Deborah knowing me well enough, I decided to 'up my gain' by messing around with her.

By feeling more confident and free from 'showing my nerves', I was kissing her all over and managed to kiss her on the lips. She was 'up for some fun' and appeared very happy right from the start. It looked as if this brief experience was a change for something better, forgetting any bad experiences.

In the same year, 1977, my father died of heart failure. With Deborah teasing me when her friends were with her, including any boyfriends she may have had. I always remember one of the happiest moments of my life, this time kissing her again as she was on top form. As I was about to leave her place, she was so nice to me, that again, I could have hugged her.

Coinciding with this pleasant incident, I was in touch with the Irish family mentioned earlier. Two of whom were living in the UK including a contact, Violet.

The good thing about Violet came when she offered words of comfort that the association was helping to 'clear my head'. This however I was seeing as a compliment and more than makes up for any misgivings or arguments we had when having a 'soft spot' for her too in the late 1960s.

In the next 2½ years, I was still visiting Deborah as well as having a girlfriend, Joanne in 1977, and the year to follow, Irene (1978); by having a certain amount of feeling for these ladies, I felt unable to have any serious relationships with them.

In 1979, Deborah turned 18 and was still at home living with her family; one day as I was about to show the latest photographs I had of her, a very unpleasant episode arose following a pleasant afternoon visiting my cousin near Alexandra Palace and ahead of visiting my family in Bristol the following day.

I was feeling very romantic over Deborah and looking forward to showing her the photographs. This brief moment however was about to come to an abrupt end.

Entering Deborah's home, I saw that she was with someone. So, dumbfounded, and not knowing how to address the situation that I was in my reaction was, "What are you doing here?" Her new boyfriend, Dave failed taking it kindly to the way I was composing myself. As I was hearing him out with a few choice words, I was finding him hypothetically talking about a 'white wedding' taking place with Deborah.

Leaving for home, her mother was fine about things and felt very sorry, adding in passing, what 'a sad world' it was; by saying this, she, at no time, couldn't be any further from the truth even if she tried.

In Bristol, I felt that it spoilt my holiday, recounting to myself. "For what good I was feeling, I would have been better off staying at home."

In the aftermath of this incident, I heard voices for the first time and attempted suicide again; the second attempt I was taking a quantity of Valium tablets and putting my head in the gas oven.

Through making my presence further and sounding harsh, I felt better off trying to hang myself. The risk however is that any failed attempt could see me paralysed and/or brain damaged for life.

This episode came as I was visiting Deborah again where her boyfriend was still present. This time, pretending to be big, 'mouthing it off' and talking out loud as in the following example…

"I don't care how skint I am. If you upset this family, I will drive down and beat you up."

In passing with his threatening attitude and pretending to be a judo expert, I am saying to myself…

"If true, then I find it unbelievable coming from this character whom I perceived as 'coming over as flash'," and almost immediately I found him the most cold-hearted individual that I have ever met.

Opposite to where I lived, before moving to Dartford, I was finding out that he had an older brother. From what I was 'picking up' he was periodically absent from home.

His older brother however, always had the 'upper hand' over him and was standing for no nonsense.

At the back of my mind, I had this belief that their relationship was to last for a limited time only; my predictions however lived up to my expectations and, over a matter of weeks, things started quietening down, with Dave nowhere to be seen.

With the 'coast already clear', I visited Deborah at home and filled her in about how much I hated Dave; I also spoke about my overdose and, to follow, complimented her about the happiness given that I continue cherishing today.

Listening in, was her mother who wanted nothing more to do with me. Including my concerns when her younger daughter Karen was stabbed repeatedly and ordered to keep away from her family.

Leaving her place that night, the nostalgic period getting to know Deborah was ending.

In summarising, Deborah is constantly near to my thoughts; she was very special to the point that I felt that we were a 'good match'. In comparison to myself she was nervous and shy. These two things may have been holding her back from having too many boyfriends until later. So, reflecting the fact that seeing her having a bigger impact on me than anyone else, things appear unlikely that I would not have been here today.

In recent years, I continue having flashbacks over the bad memories of this so-called contact at the Royal. I feel that without Deborah, I could see the flashbacks getting more intense to the point of 'doing away' with myself together. So again and on a sarcastic point, it is this contact and her contribution for my ongoing mental health problem that I remain in this position. Deborah however, I must remember for providing that 'safety net' and 'taking the edge' off the painful memories with this contact.

CHAPTER FIFTEEN

MISUNDERSTANDING SOCIAL SURROUNDINGS

1. Troublesome Neighbours

Throughout my life, I had many episodes with some lacking knowledge about autism, let alone its meaning. The year 1978 coming as no exception.

Leading up to the challenging episodes, I started living independently from the age of 27 when I was offered a flat by the Council. For the first time, I had the responsibility of accomplishing things including paying my bills on time and, reporting any defects to the Council Office.

My mother, especially, was very pleased to see at last, I could 'stand on my own two feet'. She must have thought it a great achievement getting this far in comparison to my background. Earlier, I mentioned that the doctors thought that I would never read and write and, almost coinciding in this period, an ignorant parent at kindergarten interjecting to my mother to 'put me in a home' as I was supposed to be mad.

Now, beginning a new life, I knew from the start how challenging this life was going to be. Unaware however, that when I moved, two problem families were living on the estate.

Unaware who I was up against, I accepted the flat and

started settling in and, apart from the odd encounters with fellow neighbours things were peaceful. I had at least two years living peacefully on the estate before getting to know these neighbours who I felt were bad as each other. Their characters showed that they could 'turn funny' towards anyone saying or doing something out of place.

Appearing unaware of their characters, I was taking them at 'face value' before seeing 'the other side' of them ahead of getting to know them well.

One day, I was cleaning my bike and playing Elvis songs on my cassette player; I knew that both sets of families, or, their children were still into him since his passing three years previously. So perceiving me as gentle natured, it saw them taking advantage; trying to take my bike tools lying around and throwing stones before my neighbours started coming out of their flats offering their support and getting a petition together. I thought they were very courageous showing such support; the petition however was put into place and, unaware of any consequences, I signed it.

In time I was given dirty looks by one neighbour and another time, 'sounding off' – believing that I was looking directly across to his family from my bedroom window. I was about to leave the estate precinct, when from his upstairs window, he retorted…

"Had a good look!? Shall I come down there?"

Hearing this, it appeared that I was dealing with abnormal people out to do harm.

In the same period, I had a run-in with another father; this time, with a violent past. I was introduced to him by his wife and perceived him as a violent type so I chose to be silent; on leaving, I found out from his wife that he started beating her through being in his presence. As I was getting to know this man, he had something to say about the petition.

One night on my way to the local pub, I heard him calling me a 'bald-headed' f****r. I could have answered back saying, "come down here and say that" with the risk of being 'turned over.' He was the type who declined to listen to anyone upsetting his family; at the time, I could have seen his family risking eviction if being proved the instigator in harming any neighbours on the estate.

One occasion saw a 'close call'. I was off work with sciatica in early January 1981. One day, I was about to enter the estate on my pushbike when, from a distance, I saw this individual, beckoning me to come forward over a signed petition against his family and the family living opposite me. Acting sensibly, I carried on cycling into the estate and feeling lucky with him abstaining from following me.

Right from the start, I thoroughly detested this individual and had an encounter with him when I informed his wife that a neighbour told me that their kids were deprived; so, short of bothering to find out who the neighbour was, he came up to my flat and threatened to break down the door.

Shortly after this incident, on one fine sunny day, I happened to be looking out of my living room window and saw him and his brother sitting outside with his wife situated in the middle. I felt very scared, knowing full well that by entering or leaving the flat, I risked getting 'turned over'. So, I thought by defusing any misunderstanding, that generating a letter to his wife was the correct thing to do, apologising over the upset caused.

I felt that, as a psychopath with about five brothers, I could perceive him feeling secure with himself. Knowing that he could depend on them when trouble came his way.

With things passing peacefully for a certain period of time, I had no further trouble until one day when riding my pushbike. One of his kids started acting up and getting too near, resulting in accidentally knocking him over.

When his mother got to hear about the unintentional accident, she threatened to tell her psychopath of a husband to take action. I was scared to the point of trying to protect myself by positioning the wardrobes in my bedroom with the intention of barricading myself in. And, giving enough time calling the police ahead of any incident with her husband breaking down the door.

Before any threats were put into place, I called the police; on arrival, they had no issues before making our way across to the neighbour threatening her husband to take action.

Calling the police however appeared to be a waste of time, with my neighbour telling her side of the story and getting the police on their side.

Hearing the police out, they had the nerve making accusations that I deliberately knocked the kid over and finding out whether…

I had a criminal record harming children and soon finding out whether I had, and whether I needed to see a psychiatrist.

Their behaviour I thought, was appalling and many years later I found out about The Police Complaints Commission, where, if I had known about the organisation earlier I may have had a fair chance winning my case.

In addition to 'making out to be the criminal', the police were suggesting to my neighbours on taking out a court summons.

A court summons however, I felt, was more sensible compared to getting 'turned over'. I felt the neighbour threatening to get her husband to do harm, was taking a grave risk; almost inevitably, I would have tried strangling her at the earliest opportunity recovering from my injuries.

With the police leaving, I was preparing to let this incident pass; by the time the weekend had arrived, I was entering the estate with my mother and my sister Barbara and I started 'pointing out' the troublesome neighbours.

By choice, my mother intervened. In the process, one of the neighbours made an accusation that I was taking pictures of naked children. Defending my reputation, she was threatened with legal action and had to retract her accusation through the stress of her husband walking out on her previously.

Through my mother 'fighting my corner', things were quietening down; and, no summons was issued by my neighbours as well as no further trouble from either family member. Two years on, the neighbours opposite moved elsewhere; my other neighbour with the violent ex-husband, passed away and I was 'trouble-free' for many years.

However, before my imminent move, I had a downstairs troublesome neighbour saying that I was not allowed to perform any DIY in my own home. My downstairs neighbour's partner started getting involved, as I was banging in the process of putting things on the wall. Sometimes, I could hear them arguing, and he seemed reasonable enough first time round on a separate matter.

On the second occasion, I was accused of harassing his family and following his son to school. More banging and practising tapdancing steps.

With no warning, he came to my door and was trying to break it down. It appeared that with his unsuccessful attempt, he also tried gaining access to his partner's flat beneath; hearing the commotion for herself, she must have felt scared and felt unwilling to let her partner gain access.

Both of us were fortunate enough however to avoid the consequences of this horrible individual; by the time the police arrived, he had already gone. On a second occasion, he came to me threatening to 'stamp on my head' through alleging that I was upsetting his family again.

When things were passing over, I tried appeasing my neighbour beneath me, mentioning my imminent move. When I did move, my correspondence was less forthcoming, accusing the tenant at fault for 'driving me out' of my flat.

Since my move, I have heard no more from these people and hoping that they stay as far away as possible.

2. Unfair Treatment

Since leaving school I always had problems integrating with people, with hardly any friends and, often going everywhere on my own: including The Royal.

Other than meeting a female contact, Alice, it appeared that the Royal wasn't the ideal place for meeting anyone. The venue was a breeding ground for fights or having fun at one's expense.

One night a small minority were trying to take my trousers off on the dance floor. Feeling so embarrassed, looking up at the patrons looking on, I could clearly witness these lads sinking so low and enjoying their 'horse play' at my expense. As I was known to these lads, they may have perceived I had autism by the way I was coming across with the bouncers failing to intervene.

In a separate incident, I thought too that the bouncers were sinking to the level of their customers as I was being excused. Suddenly! A crowd of them came into the toilets where I started surmising that I was about to get raped. With no hesitation, I ran to the door, with one of them grabbing my jacket ripping it in the process.

On both occasions, I came to no harm, and both sets of parties must have been looking for somebody with a disability or a 'soft touch' to 'pick on'; so, as always, for anyone acting unjustly to anyone with a disability is a coward, has an unhappy home life, or, problems in their own lives.

As I mentioned above, the Royal was a 'breeding ground' for trouble, and one night I was told to 'push off' by a gang member through having a soft spot on a girl in his crowd.

Still so young, I perceived this girl as a troublemaker and perhaps 'having it in' by lying to her crowd that I was constantly staring at her. I got known by her crowd over a game of football on the local Common; the contacts were no friends and looking for one thing – trouble.

With things bad enough on my part, I started witnessing a disgraceful act at a club that I was attending. There was young lad who tried passing his girlfriend on to me. Thinking that I was 'on to something', I made an effort talking to her before trying to ask her out and, obviously, she turned down my request.

Things however started turning nasty when I was informed by her boyfriend about another club that both attended and decided to pay a visit the next day.

As I entered the club, I was making enquiries of her boyfriend's whereabouts who was already at home. This time, he wasn't very forthcoming, adding that he would 'knock me to Kingdom Come' by continuing associating with his girlfriend.

At the same time, his father picked up the phone and came over very threatening; believing that I was acting stroppy. He came to the club and slapped my face.

In between and outside the 'club' social circle, it was a pleasure associating with everyone in the flats and I had many friends. The kids were happy associating with their friends and playing rounders in the enclosure until the late summer of 1972 with the atmosphere changing.

Around this time, a gang of unstable youths started congregating on the estate. Many of them I believe, coming from broken homes, beaten by their parents, or their parents were uncaring.

Some of these kids I knew; and that I was no angel myself when one of them had an older brother whom I hung around with nearly six years previously. None of the kids were 'pushovers'; even a kid of shorter size, or a little more than five feet, could still pack in a punch when defending himself when necessary.

I had many 'run-ins' with some of them hanging around on the estate, and the female contacts could be as bad. One day, I was cycling through the flats and, as I continued cycling, I came across the gang leader who continued to cause provocation. So I decided standing up for myself and succeeded in 'whacking' him in the face. He was none too pleased and I saw him looking so despondent through my actions.

By any standard, I was no born fighter and following this episode I came across three lads about to cause trouble and coming in the opposite direction. As they got near, I was trying to whack them and dodging their punches in the process and hitting out with sticks and iron bars.

Nearby was a dustbin offering some protection and proving adequate, until one of the lads successfully caught me on the head with an iron bar as I was contemplating getting out of the situation by running away. All three of them started running first, in the direction of the flats.

Following the attack, I was free from having any headaches or dizzy spells; in its place I may have damaged my back, resulting in taking time off work. So by letting this incident pass, things stayed peaceful until an episode of humiliation started to arise.

It was already autumn when suddenly, a crowd of girls shouted, "Let's beat Michael up!" and giving chase in the process. I felt so humiliated, that had things carried on for much longer I may have resorted to taking a cricket bat and whacking it over the head of anyone constantly causing harassment.

Spared from such action, a patrol service was starting up in time, ending the crowd of youths hanging around the estate; the residents living on the estate could, at last, live in peace.

At this time I was attending various venues, including the Cricketers and The Dragon Arms and getting barred from the latter for the first time.

One night, I returned to the Dragon Arms expecting it to be a normal night out until confronted by the manager and was asked to leave in the process. I was trying to find the reason, but he retorted, "Don't make me angry. Go."

I soon started feeling vexed before hearing from fellow

customers that he was barring a cross-selection for no apparent reason. So any action taken would inevitably fail, as evidence of any discrimination had to be proved. At the time, I wasn't diagnosed with autism or I may have had a chance proving my case with Citizen's Advice.

Today, the Dragon Arms is no longer trading. Since then, I had no further trouble from the venues I attended until the early 1980s.

In the 1980s, Disco was in full swing and I often attended the Eagle in Stratford. Before any discrepancy arose, I was allowed free access by a bouncer through being alone in the crowd.

Things however may have stayed in my favour with this kind bouncer remaining at the club for a longer period of time ahead of an instance arising…

One night, I saw a couple dancing erratically and decided to follow them. I was always having a partner to dance with and the bouncers or security guys were more relaxed.

As time progressed, one of the bouncers was unhappy and had doubts about allowing me access to the club; on this occasion, I was allowed access and soon came across a selection of women dancing around. I was about to join them for a dance when I was asked by the security guy to accompany him outside the club; I could see him clearly exaggerating about getting 'done over' by any of the karate guys already in the club. This I thought was nonsense and asked to leave, with a refund for the entrance fee refused.

Now no longer wanted at the club, I was putting things down as a 'lost cause'. Over time it was to be 'their loss' for barring too many Altons customers. With time progressing, I was wondering why I was bothering, writing to the local press and trying to give the club a bad name in the process.

About one year later, I returned to the club and found it virtually empty. I wasn't in the least surprised, and I was now associating at another night club called Altons.

3. Forgetting Past Troubles

Throughout the 1980s, it saw a very happy period and I felt very privileged to be part of the community. Until now and with the past bringing back unpleasant memories, at least I was able to have some respite. My autism however was getting in the way of things and I continued to be perceived as an 'oddball'.

Before getting into some of the silly things, it's good narrating some of the things taking place throughout the 1980s and beyond, starting with Alton's Night Club. By associating with Altons, the staff were more relaxed or 'laid back' and at the same time, forgetting the troubles of the late 1960s/early 1970s, which was a very upsetting time. As well as Alton's, I attended a nearby venue, The Bull.

This was a new beginning and making a change in comparison to hanging round my local area on weekends or attending West End night clubs. At the Bull, I eventually became very popular among its customers. When this happened, I was often performing where, hardly anyone else did; my popularity however started to increase through having the front, singing in front of the customers at both the Bull and eventually, Altons.

At this particular time, another 'showman' and formerly a good friend of mine, was also 'doing the rounds'. His nickname was 'Cybo'. He started the whole thing off by acting the clown at the Bull and creating a great atmosphere. I was often laughing at the things he said or did. Little realising that, through him, things were turning out for the better as many customers admired him.

Cybo however was loud and over-excited and often amusing the customers. Today, I continue looking on him as the funniest contact that I have ever met. Once, he got so drunk, that he stuck a long balloon between his legs and made sexual advances to nearby female patrons. This literally put me in hysterics and, even now I continue finding this period very funny.

Over a period of over five years, I often attended the Bull with no trouble from anyone until the Manager employed a doorman. Before I had my run-in with him, I noticed him getting funny with a selection of patrons and asking them to leave.

Though perceived as a loner, he decided on undermining my confidence through having a laugh with a female contact. So, making out to be superior, I was taken to another part of the pub to see the Manager before I was allowed to go. I was not however asked to leave and carried on trying to socialise the rest of the night as best I could.

My next visit saw him abstaining from taking the decision by forgetting the instance and was approached and told to behave myself; his exact words were…

"I hope you are going to behave yourself."

I replied, "I am behaving myself," until he got very stroppy and this time, asking me to leave and snatching a drink out of my hand.

As we were making our way towards the entrance, he had his back turned and immediately I started 'losing it' and whacked him in the face; so, 'like a bat out of hell', he immediately started kicking me, virtually all over; before doing so, I was already taking to the floor and for protection, was my jacket and a play station machine. So all I had was a cut thumb.

As he continued kicking, some punters tried holding him back and, when the opportunity arose, I ran out of the pub making my way to Altons; when the patrons let him go, he gave chase and nearby I hid in some empty garages for protection. When the coast was clear, I decided on making my way to the club and for the first time, I met the Manager, Steve, who was very kind and sympathetic and granted me free admission to the club.

When entering the club, I got myself cleaned up and, offering support, was the head bouncer, Ian, who thought that I had to go to hospital to get my thumb stitched up;

however, very soon the bleeding stopped and I was able to mingle with the patrons.

I was however unable to return to the Bull until informed by its regular DJ that the Manager sacked him through failing to turn up. When everyone left, he returned to the pub and knocked the manager out. I felt very delighted, believing that I could return with one exception – The Bull was closed for refurbishment for at least four months and renamed, Kables.

Alton's however, and in the beginning, saw periods with the atmosphere 'out of this world' on many occasions. One night, I observed many patrons having great fun, dancing with one another. Almost coinciding, I too had my own fun with a female contact and finding myself literally hugging and squeezing her. Since Betty 15 years or so previously, I have never felt so ecstatic.

The period referred to was November 1980 and, ever since, I have not witnessed any atmosphere like the one taking place that night.

At times however, I unconsciously acted eccentric (odd) as I was dancing with some of the contacts. So it would be good by 'throwing in' some examples for others to refrain from that I was accomplishing (doing) in my days of weirdness or immaturity.

As I was dancing with these contacts, I was often saying and doing things as in "you're cooool." Clapping my hands at the same time that I was dancing with them, tickling their chins and holding their hands. Sometimes the contact would say, "Can I have my hand back?" Also, I enjoyed ruffling their hair. I was often doing this as the 1980s progressed. Today and with conformities changing, I find that I am unable to get away too much with this harmless 'kink'.

Adding to the kink I have, one incident saw me asking to leave a venue through 'skylarking' around with one patron. The contact involved failed asking me to refrain from stroking her hair and told the bouncer and/or manager. Soon after, I was approached and asked to leave with a friend I was already with at the time. By generalising things, I thought the female contact involved was acting dishonourably and unable to take a joke.

With Alton's, things were different and felt I was socialising with like-minded people, refraining from getting anyone in trouble. I considered myself a "ladies man" 'back in the day' and was making up for difficult times previously. I had some good moments with the female patrons. One unforgettable instance came one New Year's Eve, kissing a female contact and at the end of the night, I 'went over the top' and recall saying…

"You've made the night for me," before literally hugging her and again feeling literally ecstatic.

Still 'over the top' were two female contacts nearby. With my head 'still in the clouds', unaware of what I was doing or saying, I shouted out loudly to them…

"I've pulled, I've pulled."

Looking on, they must have thought that I was acting 'absolutely bonkers'. Today, times remain when I can get 'carried away' with myself; so, with past unpleasant incidents arising, I felt at least able to forget the bad times in this happy period alone.

Also in the club's heyday, in the beginning, hardly any trouble existed. However, it changed its name to Chesters, when a well-known troublesome DJ was attending – with his demise coming when he was involved in a car crash.

At the time, I was trying to get into the music business. I performed my demos and this character had a reputation for taking the p**s or, taking advantage out of various people. I felt foolish when he asked me to sing with my trousers down and simultaneously, falling for his wrongdoing.

With the way he was behaving. I now believe that I should have refrained from trying to get into his record company; I had a selection of songs that I sent to his A&R contact; when hearing them for himself, he told me that they weren't his style. So, coming to my senses, I tried getting funny with the DJ and telling him what I thought of him. In passing, I was telling him that I would try making him feel small by him continuing taking advantage of my good character.

Things started turning nasty when his A&R contact was threatening and to follow, forced to apologise. The threats made however were to frighten me into submission and I felt that the only way to regain some of my lost pride was to write a letter.

My last encounter with this character came when he recounted 'Alright Bilco' (my nickname). He appeared friendly enough. However, by doing his best 'dashing my hopes' getting into the music business, I felt that I could no longer trust this character.

As time progressed, things started dwindling in the late 1980s and I was taking it upon myself to try a nearby club, Ritzy. In the four years I was there, I also had some good times and was well-received there too. I was often making a fool of myself, ruffling girls' hair and shaming myself on the DJ's tannoy singing out of tune and, most daring of all, going around the dance hall saying suggestive things to female contacts that I shouldn't have been saying. Today, behaving in that way is asking to be barred from many venues.

In this same period, I had my share of 'run-ins'. One of them was with a bouncer who I nearly got beaten up by, through trying to steal his girlfriend away from him. He soon however was sacked through beating up a patron.

When things started 'drying up' at the Ritzy, I felt compelled moving on elsewhere. This time getting into further trouble.

4. A Handful Of Undesirables.

With no choice moving on, I was taking my social life to the now, defunct Chestnut Tree. So, in my early 40s and still unable to socialise with anyone nearer my age, meant getting in with the wrong clientele and getting into trouble. Also, I fell short of a diagnosis for autism until 47.

At first, I was accepted and each week were karaoke sessions taking place. Little knowing however that many troublemakers often used the pub and thinking nothing better than making themselves look superior.

I soon became known by taking part in the sessions and the first I knew of any problems was when told to 'f**k off' by a foul-mouthed lad. Little realising however that many of the lads were taking exception through allegedly giving the female punters performing at karaoke, 'funny looks'. I was often trying to find out the reasons for their grievances and through being informed earlier, I may have tried addressing my conduct.

In between were good moments and one Christmas saw one of my best on record following a turbulent year with stomach pains through contracting a condition called cholecystitis (gallstones). So when told to 'f**k off' (as mentioned) this uncalled-for remark failed to dampen my spirits. However, the turning point came when I had to leave the pub together.

With karaoke returning, following a lengthy break, I started getting more aggravation and called a few choice names. Including, 'pervert', 'sex case', 'sex case hang him, hang him'. One member of the crowd however started getting very nasty and threatening, that it resulted in moving away from them to another part of the pub. Little knowing however and eventually told by some associates on my side, that by any of these lads 'ganging up', they would have taken action. By knowing 'first hand' of this protection in place, this may have resulted by staying at the Chestnut Tree longer.

However over a six-year period, I was able to return to the pub to find things changing for the better. I felt that I was now unable to get into the 'in crowd' of people through them being the wrong clientele.

In between 1994 and 1999, I decided on returning to visiting the clubs I had attended. This time however, I was in dispute with the bouncers at one of the clubs, through messing around with my car and through trying to show me up. Things however were to resolve themselves when the owner of one of the clubs passed away and I was asked to attend his funeral.

At the wake itself, my past grievances were soon forgotten and my most recent communication came when telling an elderly contact still working, that I had autism. So perhaps by learning more about the condition, he may have ended up feeling guilty whenever he started messing around with me and perhaps, other patrons with a soft touch.

So, ending my 'roller coaster' of events taking place. My social life was continuing on an even par from 2000 onwards until moving to in May 2003.

APPENDIX

On the following pages are reports backing up my mental health condition following the misunderstanding of autism in my early years. Hardly anyone knew about the condition and so, consequently I was made to fend for myself, or, might have been locked away in a mental institution for many years had it not been family intervention.

Any information on the psychiatrists' reports on the following pages, should help various professionals understand better, why so many individuals with autism end up with mental health issues.

To start with, the journey begins at Hospital. Supporting me was my sister, Josephine trying to find out whether any autistic specialist services existed in my local area; had any existed, then inevitably it would be beneficial for anyone on the autistic spectrum.

So far and by taking my current medication and undergoing past cognitive therapy, nothing much has changed referring to the following mental health conditions:

Anxiety and depression
Experiencing highs and lows

Flashbacks
Hearing occasional voices
Occasional disorientation or wandering around in a daze
Seasonal Affective Disorder (SAD) in the winter months

The latter however is relieved by light therapy. A special lamp or light box used for this purpose.

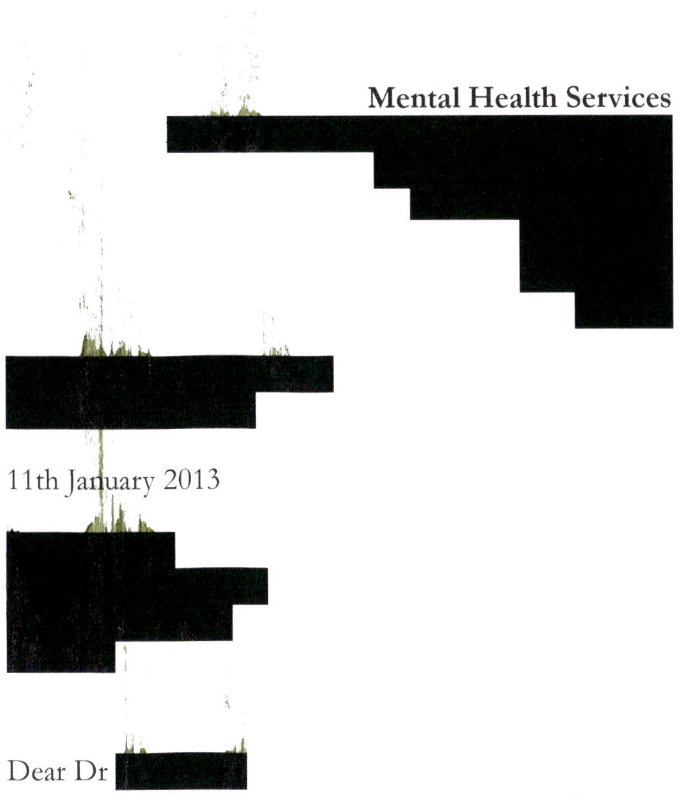

Mental Health Services

11th January 2013

Dear Dr

Re: **Mr Michael FELDMAN dob**

Date of Clinic appointment:	10.01.13
Diagnosis:	High Functioning Autism
Current problems:	Low mood, anxiety, social communication difficulties, flashbacks.

Changes to Care Plan: (Senior Social Worker, RAAT) will carry out an ADL Assessment at home next week. Unfortunately psychology services cannot offer him any therapy due to lack of specialist services that deals with autism.

GP action requested:	Continue on same medication.
Current Medication:	Citalopram 20mg mane.
Risk alerts:	Vulnerability
Relapse Indicators:	Low mood, anxiety, social isolation, flashbacks of the past events.
Crisis Plan:	To contact
Next Appointment	31.01.13 at 11am with
Contact Person	

Summary of Interview

I reviewed Mr Feldman on 10.01.13 at and Assessment Team. (Social Worker) was also present for a brief period.

He reported feeling low and anxious. He feels tearful and gets flashbacks of past events and worries about his mother who is in a nursing home. Before Christmas, he had recently been having frequent headaches and also, let down by the Day Centre by not being considerate towards him and therefore, stopped going there. He also told us that one of the ladies at the Day Centre accused him of calling her a 'bitch'. He feels isolated and does not think that he can manage on his own. However, he is able to go out and do his own shopping and manage his own finances.

Mr Feldman also gets very anxious in unfamiliar situations and has difficulty communicating with others. He can however cook meals and look after himself but, at times, struggles. He has spoken to the Samaritans when feeling desperate but denied any suicidal thoughts. He takes his medication regularly and is not keen by asking his doctor to increase the dose of the medication that he is currently taking.

His family is not happy that he is not getting the support he needs either from psychology or social services. They want him referred to the Specialist Psychology Team at Maudsley Hospital.

On mental state examination, he was casually dressed as a 62 years Caucasian gentleman who appeared slightly unkempt. He maintained good eye contact and was able to establish rapport. He appeared very anxious initially and also when he could not communicate something. His speech was normal in affect. No evidence of formal thought disorder or perceptual abnormality. His cognition is grossly intact and insight present.

I have explained to him that ████ will arrange to see him at home and that he should let his sisters know about the home visit. Referral to the Specialist Psychology Team will be discussed in a subsequent appointment with Dr ████ (Consultant Psychiatrist).

Yours sincerely

████

CC. M Feldman

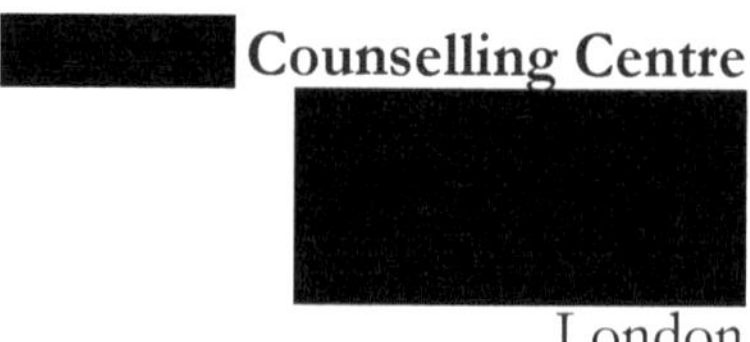
Counselling Centre

London

Dr

Dear Dr

Re: Mr Michael Feldman

Thank you for referring the above patient. Mr Feldman attended his assessment session and presented as extremely anxious and said he is finding it difficult to manage his stress levels at present and feels 'very down'. He said he has great difficulty communicating, is lacking confidence, is unable to relax, has difficulty sleeping and constantly fears rejection. He informed me that he is autistic and has had to live with being labelled 'stupid' until he was diagnosed with autistic tendencies in 1998.

Mr Feldman said he has suicidal thoughts and is frightened that he 'might do something'. He said he has taken tablets on a few occasions in the past after specific incidents, when he feels rejected, or when he gets upset about somebody else's loss – he said he lost his father in 1977 and his younger sister in 2001.

Mr Feldman also informed me he has recently been hearing voices again (he recalled hearing voices 31 years ago when he felt rejected and said he took a few tablets then). He was unable to remember what the voices said to him, but described them as 'direct voices' and said they frightened him. He also said he has bad memories of the past which he referred to as 'flashbacks' and these included feeling rejected by a lady he was fond of and someone he knew being stabbed.

Mr Feldman said he lives alone, but has relatives including his mother and two sisters, and also six friends. He informed me he is unable to work, but enjoys photography which he taught himself – he said he has now learned that it is unacceptable to take photographs of people without asking them first. He said he has had a few close relationships, but called himself 'too choosy' and attends a day centre with patrons who have similar mental health problems.

Due to the longstanding, complex nature of Mr Feldman's difficulties and the element of risk involved, I am referring him back into your care and would recommend an urgent referral to CRT (CMHT) plus a referral to Learning Disability NHS & Local Authority [redacted], who offer long-term help for adults on the autism spectrum.

Many thanks for your help in this matter.

Yours sincerely

[redacted] MBACP (Accred)
COUNSELLOR

Community Health and Social Care –

Summary of Assessment

I reviewed this gentleman on the 15th May 2017 in the outpatient clinic at Community Health and Social Care – , with his sister

This 66-year-old man was referred by his GP for depression. This was a seven-year history, worse since December 2016. He thinks that this may have been precipitated by his best friend having many social and housing problems in December. His friend was admitted to and this was a stressful time for both of them.

His 'depression' is episodic and lasts up to a week. At these times he feels flat in mood. He also reports having 'flashbacks' which he described as bad memories of specific social events. They all seem to be about the same events, surrounding interpersonal relationships. These have led him to adopting avoidance as a coping strategy. He avoids people with mental health issues. His sister explains that he has had interactions with unpleasant people in his life. The most recent issue was only this weekend. His sister went on to explain that he has always ruminated on social interactions and these thoughts tend to consume him. She also felt that he had some problems with communication. She thinks his problems are lifelong and not just in the last seven years. They relate to his way of thinking and she thought he may benefit from specialist talking therapy. He has since sought out a private psychotherapist and has had four sessions.

His sleep has been poor the last few nights due to ruminating on a recent social stressor. He has frequent micturition, up to ten or twenty times a night. He is only getting five to six hours of sleep in total; he makes up for this by napping during the day. His appetite is good and he enjoys his food. His energy is good in the mornings but he becomes more tired throughout the afternoon. I pointed out that this was very common in most people! His motivation and concentration are both good.

Past Medical History

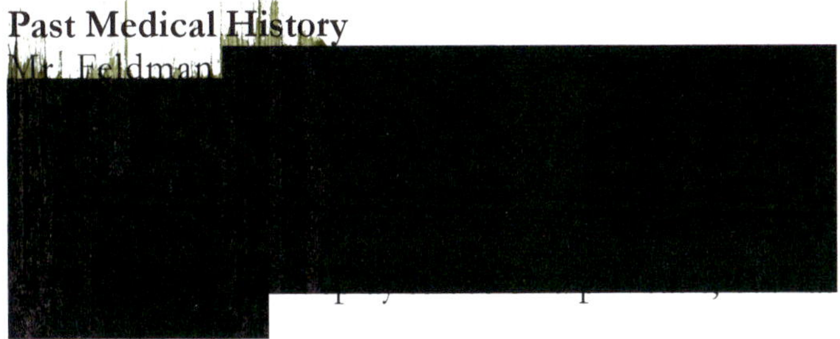

Psychiatric History

1959 – Admitted to The Maudsley due to behavioural difficulties and eating problems.

1973 – He was seen in St. Clement's outpatients. Took an overdose the day after being shunned by a girl that he was fond of, at a dance.

1979 – He had a second overdose and also attempted to gas himself.

1998 – He was seen in The Maudsley Hospital and diagnosed with high-functioning autism.

2012–2013 – He was seen in Outpatients at and saw Dr R. He also saw a psychologist at this time.

Investigations

Family History

His father died in 1977 from sudden cardiac death. His grandfather and all of his uncles had heart disease. He lost his mother two years ago from Alzheimer's disease. His sister Barbara died six years ago from an arteriovenous malformation haemorrhage. His sister Josephine is 56 and lives locally, she is well. His sister Norma is 69 and lives in Bristol, she is also well.

Personal History

Mr Feldman reports a normal birth. He did however have numerous illnesses in the first three months of life, including whooping cough, pneumonia and gastroenteritis. His mother felt he was developing slowly and he did not speak until he was 5 years old. He was always hyperactive as a child they were unaware of his diagnosis of autism in those days. His mother was only 22 years old when he was born and he describes the home environment as very stressful. He had many difficulties and was always "getting up to mischief". He had to attend a special school due to his behavioural difficulties, which was a boarding school in . He reports that the staff used to hit him and it was overall a generally unpleasant experience. After that he lived in for much of his life.

Social History

Mr Feldman currently lives at , an extra-care sheltered accommodation. He mixes less these days and says that the food is not good anymore since they changed the variety of their menu. He enjoys living there. He enjoys photography, socialising and using the computer and the internet. He is able to concentrate and enjoy all of his activities. He goes to a church in with a luncheon club. He is Jewish but he goes to churches for the social aspect.

Mental State Examination

Mr Feldman was a tidy and appropriately dressed Caucasian gentleman. He mobilised independently. There was good eye contact and rapport was established. There was some mild psychomotor agitation. His speech was normal in volume and tone and was spontaneous. There was some hesitancy and stuttering. His mood was "up and down" but his affect was reactive. He was able to reminisce happily with smiling and laughing. His thoughts were normal in form, stream and possession. There was some rumination on social events which seems to be a lifelong trait. There was some hypochondriasis but he was easily reassured. His thoughts were very positive. He denied any thoughts of deliberate self-harm or suicide. His cognition was not formally assessed but he had good recollection of recent events and he was well orientated with excellent chronological memory of life events. His insight was moderate and he was able to accept the outcome of the consultation and the recommendations. He does not smoke or drink alcohol.

Impression

There was no evidence of any severe and enduring mental illness. He has high-functioning autism and has a lifelong tendency to take socially stressful events to heart and to ruminate on these, which can affect his mood for short periods of time. He is currently having private psychotherapy and I have encouraged him to continue with this.

We also discussed his antidepressant. He is taking Citalopram 20mg but the dose was 30mg around Christmas time. I have advised him of the cardiac side-effects of doses higher than 20mg. It may be worth reducing and discontinuing his Citalopram and giving him a trial without this as his affective instability is part of his autism and not due to a major depressive disorder. If he does require an antidepressant in the future then

Mirtazapine may be a better option, to target his sleep. I have also given him some healthy lifestyle advice and have explained to him that he will be discharged back to primary care today.

Please do not hesitate to contact me should you wish to discuss this gentleman.

Yours sincerely

[REDACTED]
Consultant Psychiatrist
[REDACTED] **Older Adults Mental Health Team**

Lightning Source UK Ltd.
Milton Keynes UK
UKHW020945090922
408551UK00006B/318